YOUR HEALING HANDS

Your healing hands

DR JERZY GEORGE DYCZYNSKI

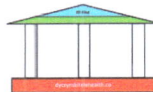

CONTENTS

Dedication - ix

~1~

Introduction

1

~2~

Reflexology

9

~3~

Workings of the foot reflexology

17

~4~

Practice of reflexology

25

~5~

Self treatment

29

~6~

Hand reflexology

35

~7~

Tale of kids' reflexology

43

~8~

Kids reflexology

51

~9~

Parents guide to kids reflexology

55

~10~

Kid's hand reflexology

57

~11~

Reflexology of the kids forearms

65

~12~

Long moves of reflexology

71

~13~

Your sequence of kid's reflexology

75

~ 14 ~

Ear reflexology

83

~ 15 ~

Reflexology with the feet

87

About the author - 89
Acknowledgements - 93

This book is dedicated to all fitness Enthusiasts and holistic health Seekers. This book "Your healing hands. The power of reflexology" has a clear, consistent and accurate message for you. Just do it.

This book is for the young generation of the 21st century. It addresses the modern families and their kids.

~ 1 ~

INTRODUCTION

A man suffering from a dreaded skin disease came to Jesus, knelt down, and begged him for help. If you want to, he said, you can make me clean. Jesus was filled with pity, and reached out and touched him. I do want to, he answered. Be clean! At once the disease left the man, and he was clean. Mark Chapter 1, Verse 41-43.

The use of hands for healing and therapeutic purposes—such as touching, massaging, laying on of hands, and anointing with oil—has a long and rich history. These practices date back over 2000 years before Christ when Abraham lived between the Euphrates and Tigris rivers in Mesopotamia, a region that now includes parts of modern-day Iraq and Palestine. Healers in ancient India, China, and Egypt also employed these methods. The Greeks and Romans embraced these healing practices as well. This rich heritage connects us to a long-standing tradition of healing that encompasses reflexology, spanning centuries.

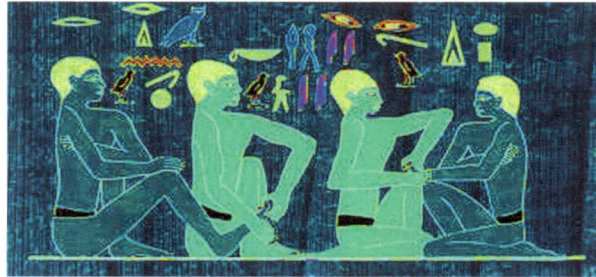

**Picture 1. Massage and reflexology in ancient Egypt.
Wikipedia.**

This ancient wall painting is located in the tomb of Ankhmahor, the highest official after the Pharaoh, often referred to as the physicians' tomb. The painting illustrates the practice of foot and hand reflexology, a form of healing therapy that focuses on pressure points in the hands and feet. It dates back to 2330 BC (Before Christ).

The historical context of massage and reflexology can connect you to a long-standing tradition of healing with human hands, fostering a sense of continuity between conventional medicine and natural healing practices. Your understanding of the proven benefits of these therapies, supported by scientific evidence, can provide reassurance to you and your friends regarding their effectiveness.

Reflexology applies gentle pressure to the feet and hands, functioning similarly to acupuncture by using entry points that access the body's energy channels. Both reflexology and massage aim to promote relaxation, relieve stress and tension. Reflexology is amazing in the improvement of your emotional and intellectual well-being.

Reflexologists hold a deep understanding of the body's energy channels and use specific points on the hands and feet that correspond to various organs, effectively connecting with the body's energetic systems. The traditional medicine approach to reflexology and massage therapy has been passed down through generations and is supported by scientific evidence highlighting its benefits. Reflexology, which includes touching, rubbing, or kneading the body's soft tissues, helps relax the nervous system by lowering the heart rate and blood pressure. It also balances stress and pain hormones while enhancing immune function.

Reflexology technique can be applied using the hands, fingers, elbows, knees, forearms, or even the entire feet.

In reflexology, a kid's hand holds special significance. It acts as a unique connection to the internal organs, providing valuable insights into the 's health and well-being for knowledge-able reflexologists or parents. During early development, kids use their hands to explore and comprehend the external world since their vision is not fully developed until they are several months old or even up to a year.

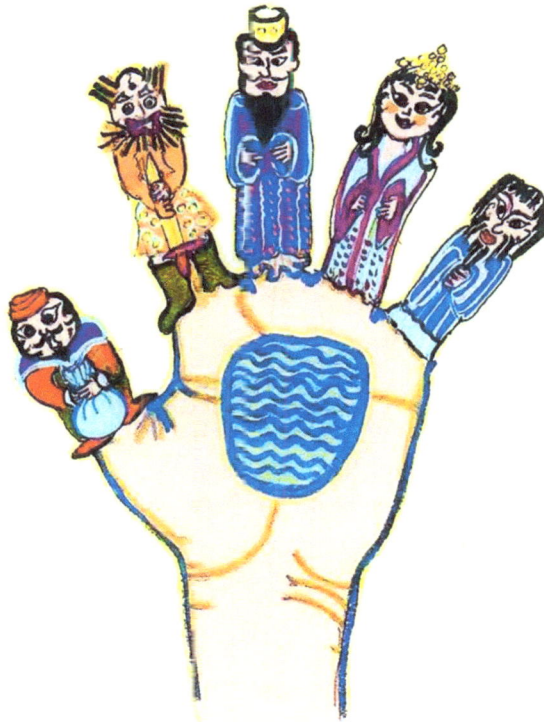

Picture 2. The kid's hand has a traditional medical connection to the internal organs. Courtesy Angela Rudhart-Dyczynski.

According to traditional medicine, fingers are not just digits; they represent miniature versions of vital organs. The middle finger, known as the "king," corresponds to the heart. The fourth finger, or "queen," is linked to the lungs. The fifth finger, referred to as the "healer," embodies the kidneys and adrenal glands, highlighting their high curative potential. The index finger, called the "general," has a reflective connection to the gallbladder and liver. Finally, the thumb, known as the "minister of supply," corresponds to the digestive system, including the spleen and stomach.

A fundamental aspect of traditional reflexology for kids is the connection between specific areas of the hand and the developing internal organs. Gentle, safe techniques used in children's reflexology include pressing and rubbing the fingers and making circular movements on the kid's hands to tap into the vital energy center, like a lake located in the middle of the kid's palm.

Reflexology techniques for children often involve quicker movements than those used for adults. The speed at which reflexologists apply these techniques corresponds to the child's age and natural heartbeat rates. For example, newborns typically have an average heartbeat of 130 to 180 beats per minute. A one-year-old child's heart rate ranges from 90 to 150 beats per minute, while a two-year-old averages about 90 to 130 beats per minute. Three-year-old children generally have an average heart rate of around 100 beats per minute, and children aged six to eight typically average about 90 beats per minute.

Reflexology is an effective method for reducing bodily stress and relieving muscle tension. It works on a deeper level by restoring the functionality of ligaments and cartilage, alleviating pain, and promoting intellectual growth as well as emotional well-being. Reflexology sends impulses through energy channels connected to major nerve pathways and internal organs, offering holistic healing that goes beyond merely addressing physical symptoms.

In European countries, individuals professionally trained in reflexology and massage are traditionally referred to as masseurs (for males) or masseuses (for females). In the United States, the gender-neutral term "massage therapist" is more commonly used, while in some provinces of Canada, practitioners are known as registered massage therapists. Although reflexology and massage therapy share similarities and offer benefits, each serves a distinct purpose and requires specialized training. Massage therapists are usually trained and have great skills in reflexology.

Reflexology is an alternative medical practice that is grounded in scientific principles. It involves applying pressure to specific points on the hands, feet, and ears, which promotes relaxation. The techniques used in reflexology include rubbing with the thumb, fingers, and hands. The mechanical impulses generated by reflexologists are converted through collagen fibers into electrical signals that travel along the nerves to reach your brain.

Intriguingly, the entire body is represented in your brain, often referred to as the "homunculus," or "petite man."

You can think about it as a three dimensional hologram placed between two hemispheres, left and right part of your brain. This small mini hologram represents your miniaturized body within your brain.

Conversely, the body itself, including the brain, is also mapped onto the hands, feet, and ears. These sensory organs are uniquely connected to the brain to collect impulses and information.

In reflexology, specific areas associated with the body are stimulated by applying pressure. This pressure mimics the body's natural connections with its environment. The hands of reflexologists send impulses to the corresponding body parts represented in the brain's homunculus. These interactions promote effective communication between the reflective organs and the brain, which is essential for maintaining overall health.

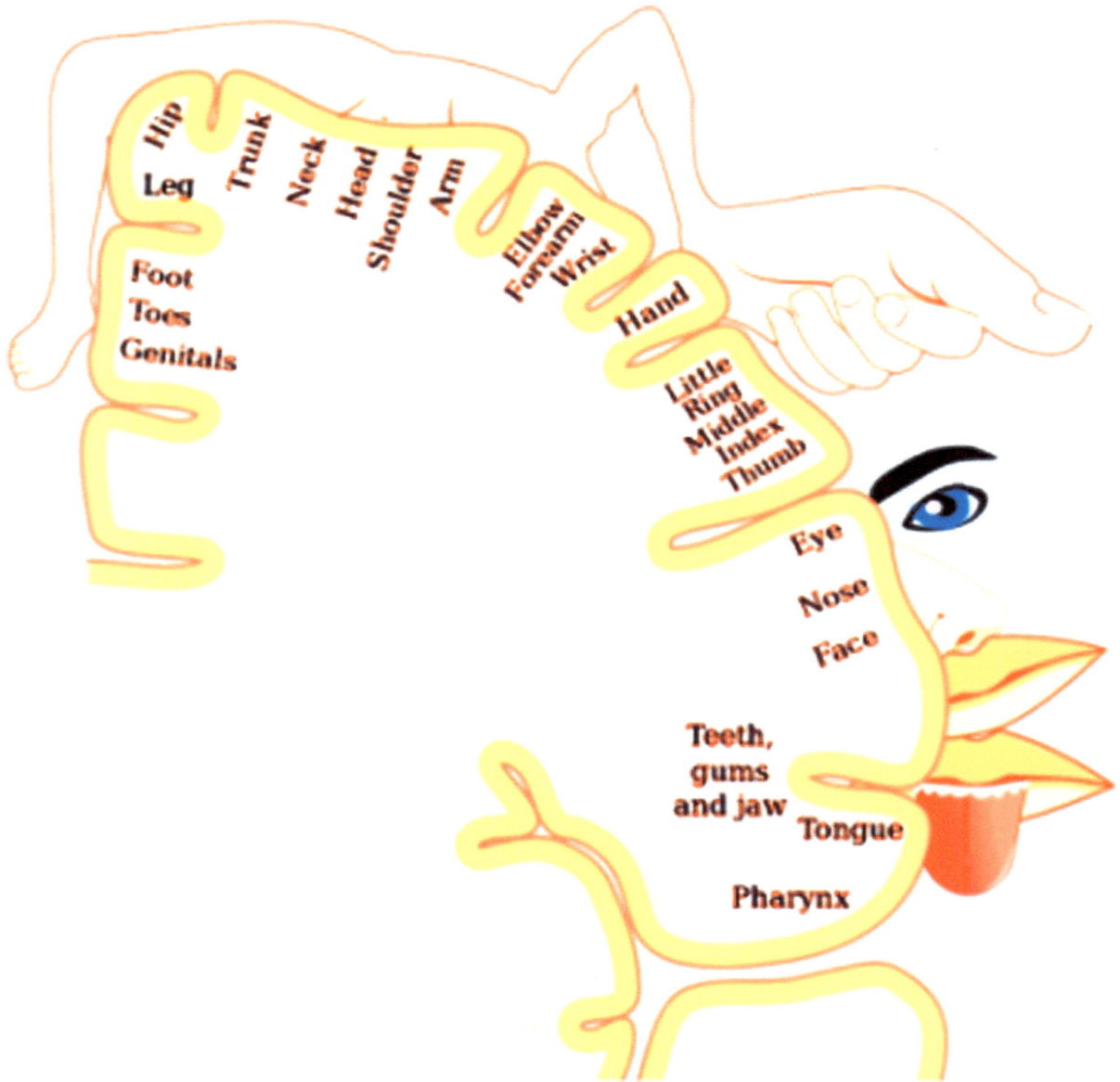

Picture 3. Small man in the brain. Wikipedia.

The feet, hands, and ears act as a mini hologram of the entire body, facilitating communication with your surroundings, nature, and other people. In reflexology, this "hologram" refers to the miniature representations of the entire body that can be found on the hands, feet, and ears. These sensory body parts are constantly in contact with the environment. For instance, the ears, which detect and interpret sounds, play a vital role in this process.

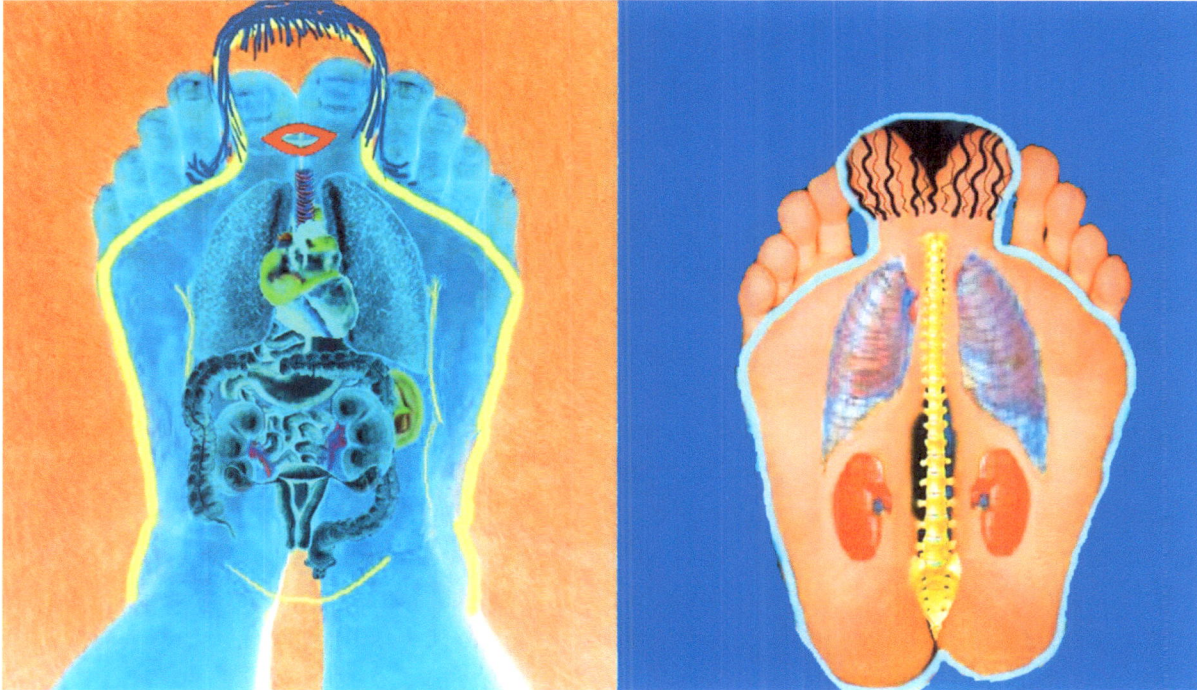

Picture 4. Hologram of the body in the feet, front and back view.

Your feet have a solid connection to the earth's soil. Similarly, your hands play a dual role in making contact with your environment and the people around you, such as family, friends, and neighbors, making them vital for your body's sensory connections. The critical difference is that reflexology is generally performed only on the feet, hands, and ears. In contrast, massage therapy can be performed on any body part.

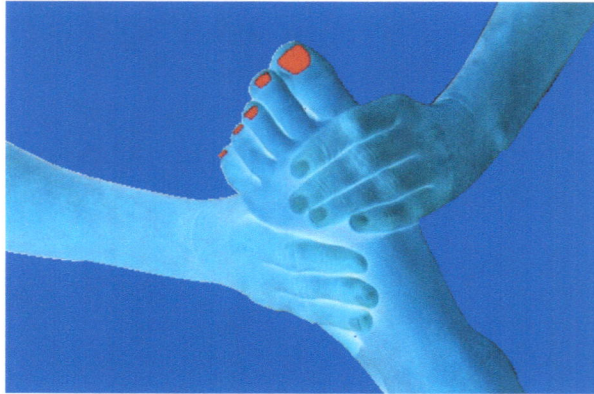

Picture 5. Foot reflexology.

Medical reflexology is a specialized therapy aimed at addressing specific symptoms such as pain, strain, or defined medical conditions. It includes the application of mechanical impulses, which are controlled and measured. The pressure or force applied to the skin and connective tissue invoke a response. These impulses and responses help the body adapt to changes and activate its self-organizing capabilities, resulting in a range of benefits.

Clinical reflexology is a versatile approach that combines various styles and techniques, including bioenergetics. It is not confined to a single method, allowing for a personalized experience. Reflexology can be applied to the foot, ear, and hand, utilizing the reflective areas found in these regions and the energy channels within the body. Activating the entry points to these energy channels is essential in reflexology. A skilled therapist plays a vital role in identifying and correcting imbalances in your body's energy flow. By considering your unique situation and medical history, the reflexologist can tailor their methods to meet your specific needs. This customized approach promotes relaxation, enhances overall well-being, and provides relief from muscular and pain. It also improves the flexibility of your joints.

~ 2 ~

REFLEXOLOGY

The eye cannot say to the hand, I don't need you! And the head cannot say to the feet, I don't need you! 22 On the contrary, those parts of the body that seem to be weaker are indispensable, 23 and the parts that we think are less honorable we treat with special honor. And the parts that are unpresentable are treated with special modesty. Corinthians Chapter 12, Verse 21-23.

For over 5,000 years, feet have been valued for their healing properties as reflective organs. Foot reflexology is a universal healing practice historically significant among Native Americans, Egyptians, and Incas. This rich tradition has also developed in Europe, India, and China.

Passed down through generations, the global practice of reflexology fosters a deep sense of connection to natural healing. It creates a feeling of belonging among those who have experienced its benefits and are eager to share their positive experiences with foot reflexology.

Reflexology is based on the ingenious design of your body. Each internal organ is uniquely connected to the external environment through the eyes, feet, hands, and ears—organs that gather essential information for optimal functioning of the WHOLE, which is more than just the sum of its parts.

This complex interaction showcases the sophistication of your amazing body.

The feet play an influential role in this process, as they can sense the texture, temperature, and consistency of the ground. More than 100 specific areas on the feet are connected to internal organs through 40,000 nerve fibers, which transmit signals via the spine, brain, solar plexus, and pelvic plexus. Is it not amazing? This sensory information is relayed to these centers and directed to the corresponding internal organs.

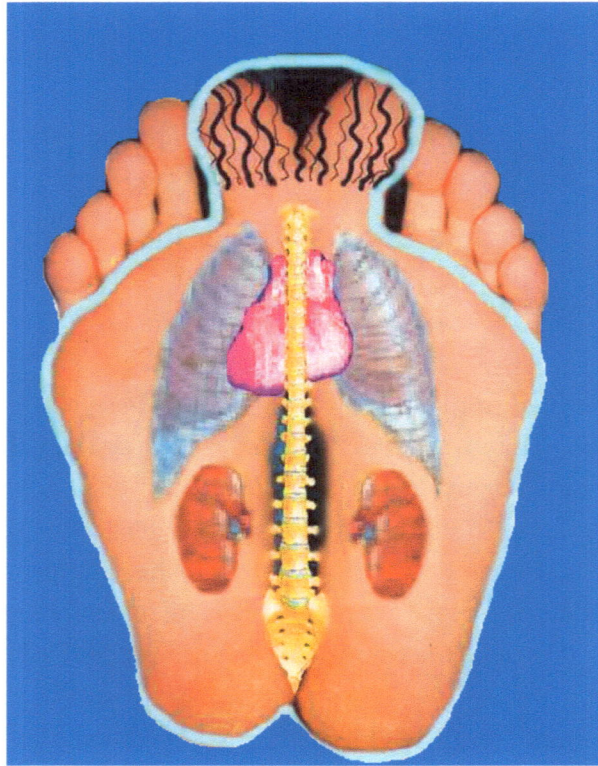

Picture 6. Mini representation of the organs in the feet.

Touch and tactile sensors in our hands enable us to engage with the world around us and connect with family and friends. Our ears are equipped with sensors that detect airwaves, sounds, and vibrations, which play a vital role in both our internal and external communication.

Reflexology is grounded not just in theory but in the meticulous research of Dr. William H. Fitzgerald, a medical doctor and ear, nose, and throat (ENT) specialist. In 1913, he developed a scientifically based framework for reflexology. His work, along with contributions from Miss Eunice Ingham in the United States and reflexology therapist Hanne Marquard in Germany, established the scientific foundation for reflexology. Dr. Fitzgerald's research was groundbreaking in the fields of reflexology and bioenergetic medicine. He explored the invisible energy channels that run through the body, referred to as meridians in traditional Chinese medicine. His findings provided a scientific basis for reflexology, illustrating the complex networking among the body's various systems and internal organs. Dr. Fitzgerald discovered that the body is unified by ten energy channels that extend from the tips of each finger and toe to the head, and vice versa. Stimulating energy flow in one area of a channel creates a ripple effect, influencing the entire channel and its associated internal organs.

Reflexology is based on several key principles. The foot, ear, and hand are external sensory organs that contain miniature representations, or holograms, of the entire body and its parts. These mini representations of internal organs act as mirrors, reflecting the body's internal functional state.

For instance, if there is a problem with your liver, it will send signals to the feet, particularly to the area that corresponds to the liver. As a result, that particular area may become tender or even painful. This tenderness can be felt not only in the corresponding area on the surface but also in the deeper structures beneath it, leading to discomfort of the soles while walking.

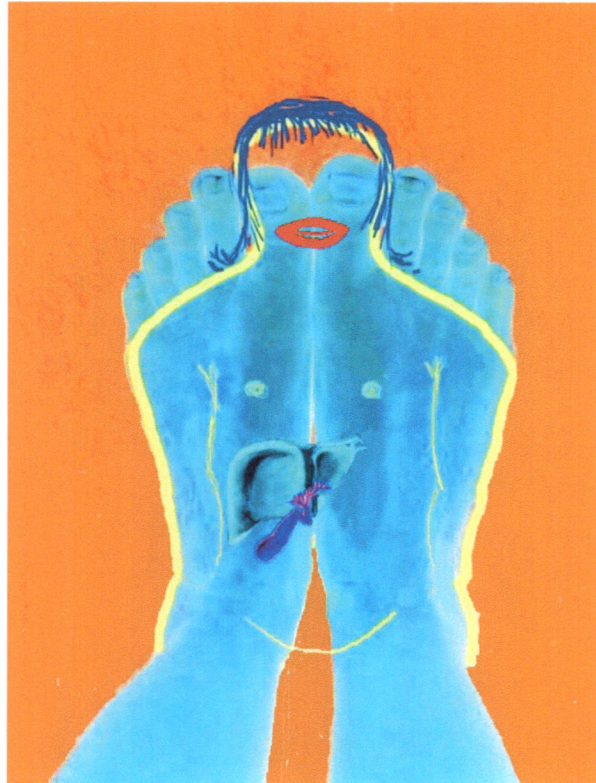

Picture 7. Mini hologram of the liver in the feet.

Feet have also a reasonable amount of entry points for the energy channels that traverse the entire body. The functions of the feet can be viewed as microcosms of the body, containing the mini representation of your body, the hologram and various entry points to energy channels that either originate from or culminate in the feet. This insight highlights the complexity and sensitivity of our feet, which are often among the most sensitive organs in your body.

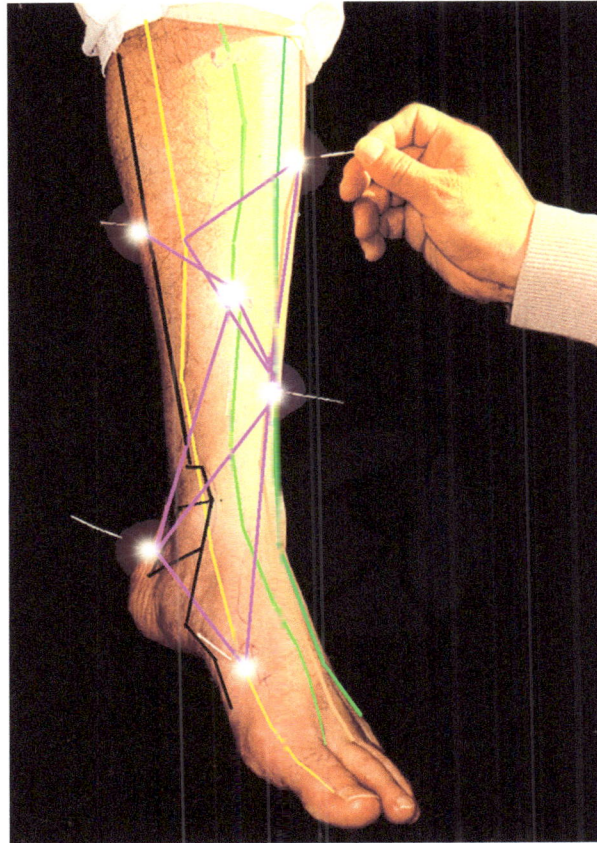

Picture 8. Energy channels with their entry points on the foot and ankle.

The reflexive areas on your feet correspond to specific organs or functions. Stimulating these reflexology areas or the entry points to the energy channels can enhance your body's functionality and help address disturbances in the internal organs, including the heart and brain.

For example, stimulating the reflexology areas linked to the head and brain can help alleviate headaches and improve intellectual clarity. Similarly, targeting the reflexology areas related to the heart can assist in managing stress and preserving good cardiovascular health.

These mini representations of internal organs in the feet, hands and ears are supported by energy channels with their regulative entry points. This collaboration creates a network that facilitates the smooth flow of vital energy throughout the body, nourishing the hands and feet with essential energy and vitality.

This holistic approach to reflexology illustrates that treating one part of the body can benefit your integrity as the WHOLE, your body as the self-organizing system.

Your body possesses an innate ability to heal itself—it is a self-organizing entity with a remarkable capacity for regeneration. After experiencing illness, stress, injury, or disease, the body may enter a state of imbalance where vital systems do not function optimally. This disruption can hinder the body from restoring its natural equilibrium, but with the right support, the body can overcome these challenges and restore its natural balance.

Reflexology, with its unique ability to detect and address these imbalances, plays a leading role in restoring natural balance and facilitating healing naturally. The reflexologist is your guide in this process. Her or his expertise will help you to navigate your body's on its healing pathway.

The application and effects of reflexology therapy are unique to each individual. The skilled, sensible hands of an experienced reflexologist , a trained practitioner who understands the body's reflective areas and their connections to internal organs, can identify imbalances, asymmetries, minor deposits, tensions, micro-injuries in ligaments, and much more. By working on specific points, the therapist helps release stagnation in the energy flow.

The reflexologist shown below applies gentle pressure with her index finger on the entry point to the liver energy channel, which is an important area for regulating liver function. Her thumb supports the pressure under the big toe. The reflexologist's finger is pressing on one of the most prominent lymphatic vessels in the foot, where immune cells can often become stagnant. Her actions help to push these cells back into the lymphatic circulation.

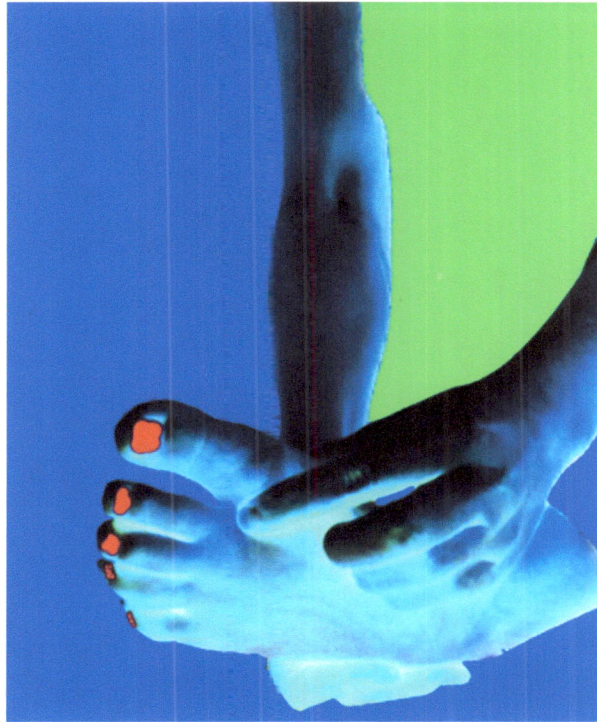

Picture 9. Foot reflexology.

Reflexology is not only a traditional healing practice; it also aligns with contemporary breakthrough discoveries such as the Biophotonic Quantum Holographic Matrix and the DNA bio-computer. These discoveries suggest a close connection between reflexology and your DNA, further validating the effectiveness of this traditional medical technique. This alignment with modern scientific science provides an additional reassurance that reflexology is a credible and natural form of therapy.

Research indicates that reflexology is a versatile therapy that can help lower systolic blood pressure and manage many symptoms. It has been shown to alleviate issues such as asthma, anxiety, headaches, migraines, postmenopausal syndrome (PMS), and even nasal congestion. By accessing specific pressure points in the feet and hands, individuals can experience relief and a renewed sense of vitality.

~ 3 ~

WORKINGS OF THE FOOT REFLEXOLOGY

I praise you, for I am fearfully and wonderfully made. Wonderful are your works; my soul knows it very well. Psalm 139, Verse 13-14.

A multitude of spiral collagen fibers, remarkable components within your body, are actively at work in your feet and hands during your daily activities. In reflexology, these fibers, along with pressure, touch, and pain receptors, function similarly to piezoelectric crystals, which generate an electrical charge in response to mechanical stress.

When mechanical pressure is applied, these fibers are squeezed and generate a current that is transmitted to the brain, enhancing communication between neurons and the treated areas of the feet, ears, or hands.

Your collagen fibers are special receptors that convert mechanical stimuli—such as pressure or touch—into electrical signals. This ongoing communication moderates your individual pain threshold. Essentially, the mechanical stimulation, which was transformed through the spiral collagen fibers into electrical impulses, travels to the brain, solar and pelvic plexus, as well as to the vagus nerve. The pattern of impulses received and interpreted by the brain and other sensory structures determines how your body interacts with the environment and how the external reality is perceived.

It is comforting to recognize that the body has the amazing ability to heal itself. Your body has an incredible capacity for regeneration. Following illness, stress, injury, or disease, the body may fall into a state of imbalance. However, reflexology can help by detecting and addressing these imbalances, guiding your body back to its natural state of balance, facilitating healing, and restoring normal functionality.

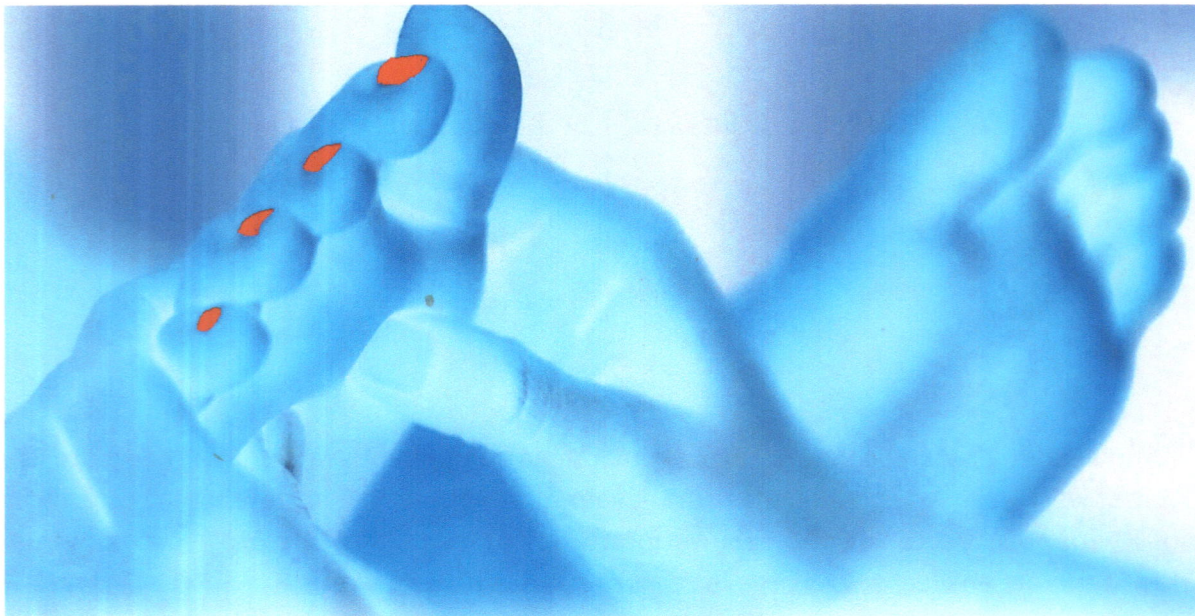

Picture 10. Foot reflexology.

The reflexologist can gently apply pressure with her fingers to specific reflective areas and entry points to energy channels located in your feet. This stimulation targets critical reflective regions associated with your heart, brain, digestive, and cardiovascular systems. The therapist senses, presses, or rubs the entry points of the energy channels that help regulate your liver, gallbladder, kidneys, spleen, and stomach functions. A special grip can be performed with the index finger on the area between the big and second toe, where the thumb cushions the pressure from underneath the toe. It regulates the liver function, counteracts the allergies and boosts the immune system.

The reflexologist's fingers also work on the lymphatic system, particularly focusing on one of the most prominent lymphatic vessels between the big and second toes. This area often experiences stagnation of immune-competent cells, preventing them from moving forward. The reflexologist helps push these cells back into the lymphatic system and blood-

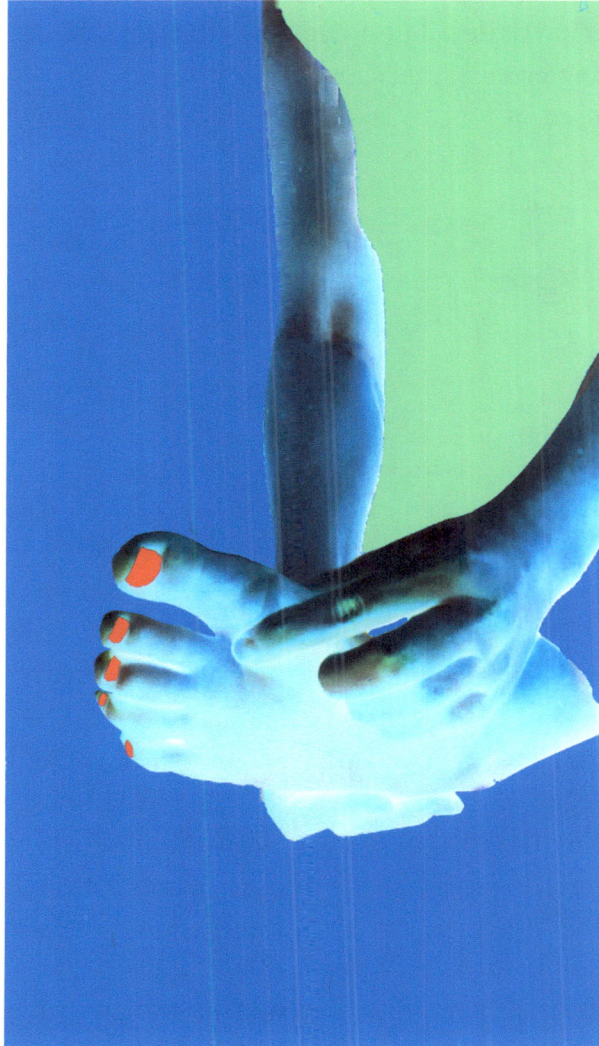

Picture 11. Foot reflexology on a lymphatic vessel.

stream by applying upward and downward pressure along this lymphatic vessel.

Foot reflexology is a therapeutic practice that includes applying pressure, rubbing, and gliding moves to the feet. It combines treatment and diagnosis. A skilled reflexologist will identify sensitive or swollen areas that correspond to your body's internal organs or part of your body. This careful attention to detail improves the effectiveness of the therapy and assures you that you are receiving professional care.

A common technique used in foot reflexology includes a technique using bent fingers or knuckles.

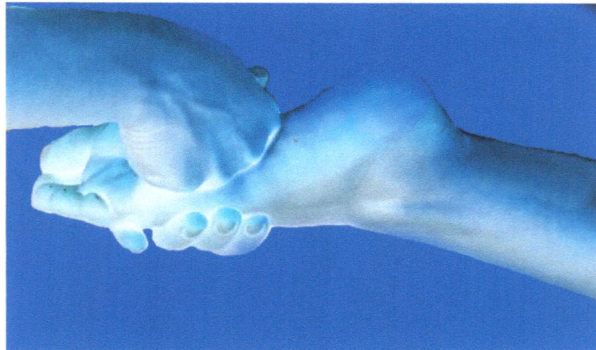

Picture 12. Foot reflexology with knuckles.

This method stimulates reflex areas and energy entry points on the feet, activating miniature representations of the organs and helping to release any blockages. As a result, waves of vital energy are generated, leaving you feeling invigorated and revitalized. Applying firm pressure on the spiral collagen fibers stimulates the brain, solar plexus, and pelvic plexus, further enhancing the flow of energy throughout your body. Foot reflexology is a technique that encourages personalization and experimentation. The following outline is just one approach to this practice, and fitness seekers are supported and encouraged to adapt and modify it to suit their specific needs.

The author has developed a simple 10-step routine for foot reflexology through years of practice.

Ten-Step Guide.

• Step One.

Establish a vital and emotional connection. Begin by applying gentle pressure around the left big toe. This connection is physical, as it relates to nerve pathways, and emotional, as it stimulates the creative right hemisphere of the brain, fostering empathy and mutual understanding.

• Step Two.

Focus on the reflective area at the base of the left big toe, which corresponds to the neck, cervical spine, and thyroid glands. Next, pay attention to the four adjacent toes that represent the sensory organs: the eyes, ears, nose, and the ethmoid bone located between the eyes, often referred to as the third eye.

• Step Three.

Target the inner side of the feet by stimulating areas linked to the spine, spinal column, and the entry points of the spleen's energy channel alongside the inner edge of the feet.

• Step Four.

Shift your focus to the outer side of the feet, addressing reflective areas associated with the urinary bladder, gall bladder, hips, shoulders, and arms.

• Step Five.

Apply repeated pressure with the thumb or knuckles to the middle of the sole. This invigorates reflective areas connected to internal organs such as the liver, heart, lungs, spleen, kidneys, digestive system, and solar plexus. This step can lead to noticeable improvements in the internal organs' functionality.

• **Step Six.**

Place your fingers between the patient's toes and apply pumping pressure to enhance lymphatic circulation. This activates entry points related to the stomach, liver, and gall bladder energy channels, increasing sensitivity in the six sense organs.

• **Step Seven.**

Perform energetic scraping of the sole with your fingers along the feet and toes. This intense stimulation feels sometimes overwhelming, but it reaches almost all reflexive areas and promotes energy flow throughout the body.

• **Step Eight.**

Conclude with gentle gliding moves using your fingertips along the ankles, shins, calves, and feet. This aligns the reflective areas with the entry points of the energy channels. Use gentle circular motions on the foot and ankle to connect the flow of vital energy between the energy channels and the reflective areas that correspond with various organs.

• **Step Nine.**

To reinforce the kidney channel's origin point at the center of the forefoot, hold the middle of the foot gently between your hands, focusing on the first kidney entry point until you feel the gentle waves of vital energy emerge.

• **Step Ten.**

Communicate with your patient, client, or friend your observations concerning the strengths of pulsations, areas of exceptional sensitivity, and your impression of the general health of the person you have treated with reflexology.

Foot reflexology adopts a holistic approach to wellness. By stimulating the soles of the feet, you engage all the organs, particularly those associated with the kidney channel, providing comprehensive treatment. This holistic method ensures that every related body part is addressed. The suggested foot reflexology sequence comprises ten steps designed for specific purposes and techniques. However, every reflexologist can tailor their methods to meet individual needs, drawing on their observational skills, touch diagnostics, insights, and experience.

~ 4 ~

PRACTICE OF REFLEXOLOGY

The reflexologist begins by gently touching your feet with fingers, creating a sense of relaxation. Then, the reflexologist applies specific techniques on the reflective points, always prioritizing your comfort. Skilled reflexologists perform foot reflexology, even on feet that are highly sensitive, ensuring a comfortable and safe experience. The excellent reflexologist understands the delicate balance between discomfort and pain, ensuring that the foot reflexology is effective and creates a sufficient response, all within a relaxing and comfortable scope.

Reflexology is very popular, particularly among those dealing with chronic fatigue, degenerative knee and hip changes, and cardiovascular infirmities. Some reflexology centers can offer free treatment to encourage you to use reflexology more often. This makes this holistic, ancient practice accessible to all. After a reflexology session, you can experience a significant boost in energy, leaving you feeling invigorated and better prepared to tackle the challenges of modern life.

Reflexology is widely recognized by holistic, sound, and experienced doctors. It provides a deeper understanding of the complexity of regulations in your body and sometimes a good explanation of the symptoms that the mini representations of your internal organs in your feet reflect your overall health. If the heart starts to fail, it can lead to poor circulation, which can manifest first as cold feet.

During your first visit, your reflexology therapist may ask general questions about your health, lifestyle, and medical history.

However, a good reflexologist will also read your feet with their skilled hands and tell you about the past major health events that have affected your life. A reflexology session usually lasts 30 to 60 minutes. You usually lie down or sit in a reclining chair for reflexology treatment. The reflexologist applies finger pressure at the reflective areas and entry points to your energy channels while guiding you on the correct breathing technique. If accidentally, the introduction of the correct breathing technique for some reason does not happen, remember that you are not just a passive recipient in your reflexology session but an active participant. Your role, especially when applying the correct breathing technique, is vital in oxygenating your brain and feet. As the reflexologist applies finger pressure at the reflective areas and entry points to your energy channels, you can actively contribute to the process and take responsibility for your breath.

One of the most efficient breathing techniques you can practice during a reflexology session is the orbital flow of breath. When used correctly, this technique can significantly enhance your reflexology experience.

When mastered, it is a powerful tool that can help you feel the energy moving in orbital breathing. This energy flow starts from the solar plexus in your lower abdomen and then raises from the end of your spine in your pelvis to the head and upper lip. This is all part of the inhalation.

When you reach the peak of your total breath intake, hold it for a second and then release your breath, exhaling and directing the energy from the lower lip to the lower abdomen and crotch. The exhalation usually lasts longer, about seven to eight seconds. This extended exhalation is not just a part of the breathing technique but also plays a crucial role in detoxifying your body at the highest possible rate, making you feel healthier and more energized.

Reflexology offers a relaxing and soothing experience, but you may occasionally feel discomfort or slight pain in certain areas. Your therapist, knowledgeable in this practice, will explain that this discomfort might be related to low-functioning internal organs or blockages in energy channels, which can impact the flow of energy in your body or specific areas. While your reflexology therapist may suggest additional sessions, many people experience significant improvement after just one treatment. This possibility for rapid and noticeable progress can instill a sense of hope and optimism as you work to enhance your health.

Reflexology is generally safe and does not typically cause many side effects. After a treatment, it is common to feel relaxed, which may lead to lightheadedness. Your feet might feel

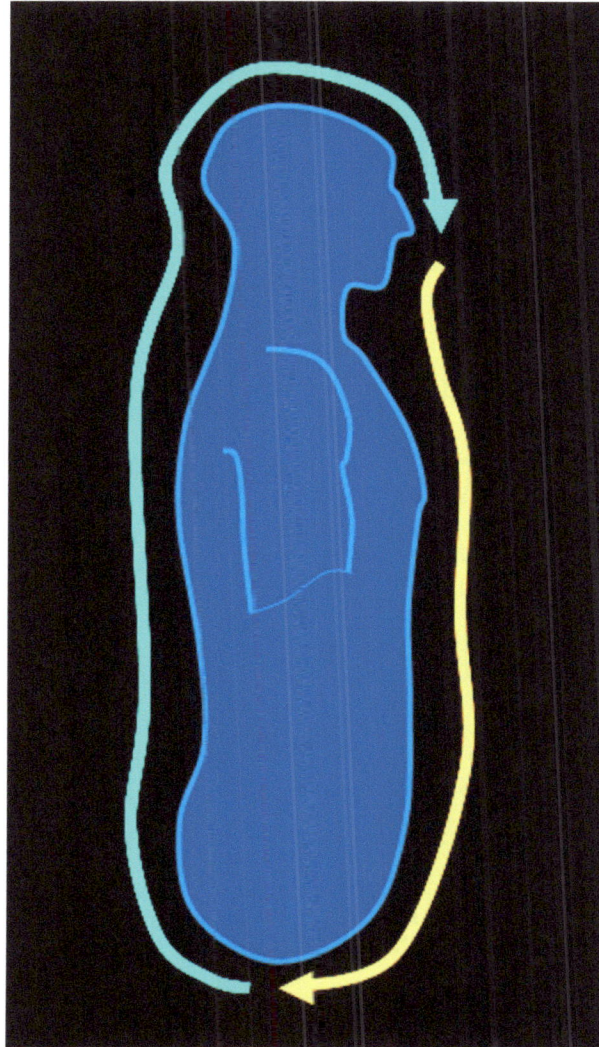

Picture 13. Microcosmic orbit by Bostjan46. Wikipedia.

tender afterward, and you may experience heightened emotions, such as feeling more emotional or tearful than usual. These reactions are normal and not a cause for concern. Additionally, you might notice that you need to pass water more frequently, which can indicate improved heart and kidney function.

To enhance the benefits of your reflexology session, it is important to stay hydrated. Consider drinking alkaline water afterward. It is advisable to avoid stimulants like caffeine, alcohol, tobacco, and recreational drugs. Instead, take some time for yourself to relax and enjoy a quiet afternoon. Following this post-treatment advice can help you maximize the benefits of your reflexology experience.

~ 5 ~

SELF TREATMENT

Jesus said to them, Surely you will quote this proverb to me. Physician, heal yourself. And you will tell me, Do here in your hometown what we have heard that you did in Capernaum. Luke Chapter 4, Verse 23.

One of the empowering aspects of reflexology is that you can apply it to yourself. Using the side of your thumb or the tip of your forefinger, you can press the desired reflective areas and the entry points to your energy channel points on your foots, hands or ears.

Maintain a pressure contact between your thumb and index finger through your foot while moving your thumb and the fingertip of your index along your foot area between the big and second toe. These two fingers will press gently up and down the lymphatic vessel lying between these two toes several times. This grip is the most important in self-applied reflexology. It boosts your immune system daily, prevents stagnation in the lymphatic vessels, improves the functionality of your liver and heart, and makes you feel more vital energy.

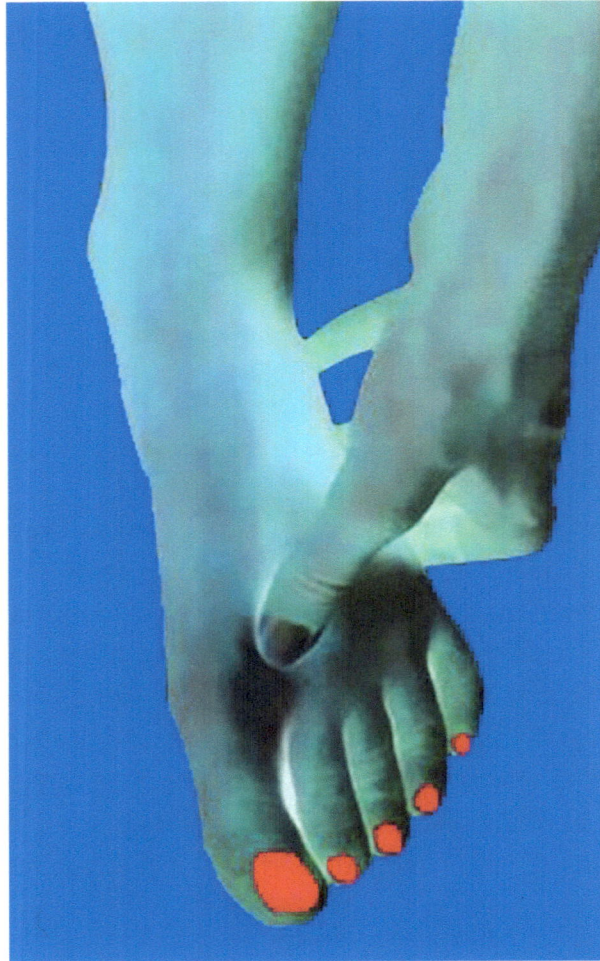

Picture 14. Self foot reflexology.

Simultaneously, you are working on the entry points to the liver energy channel, which begins between your big and second toe. This powerful synergy between the energy channels and the reflective areas on your feet reinforces your self-therapeutic actions, empowering you to make it to your daily wellness routine. As your energy channels begin or end in your feet and hands, you can treat many entry points to energy channels on your feet and hands.

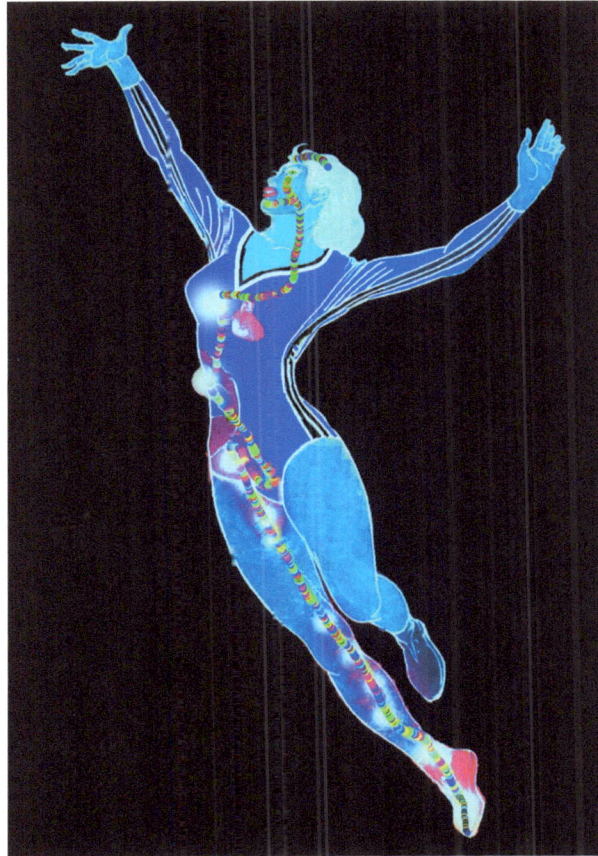

Picture 15. Liver energy channel.

Complete the reflexology of your feet with 'breeze strokes' alongside the inner curve of your foot, reflecting the course of your entire spine. This technique includes gentle strokes, as if you were creating light, frequent finger moves of the air, an energetic breeze. This helps to relax your spine and promotes overall well-being, fostering a deep connection and harmony between your body and mind.

The body can heal itself. It is a self-organizing system with a high level of regeneration. Following illness, stress, injury, or disease, it is in a state of imbalance, where vital body systems are not functioning optimally, preventing the body from restoring its natural balance and facilitating healing. Reflexology can be used to detect and address these imbalances. For instance, it can help with headaches, digestive issues, and stress. This self-applicable technique can be a powerful tool in your daily wellness routine.

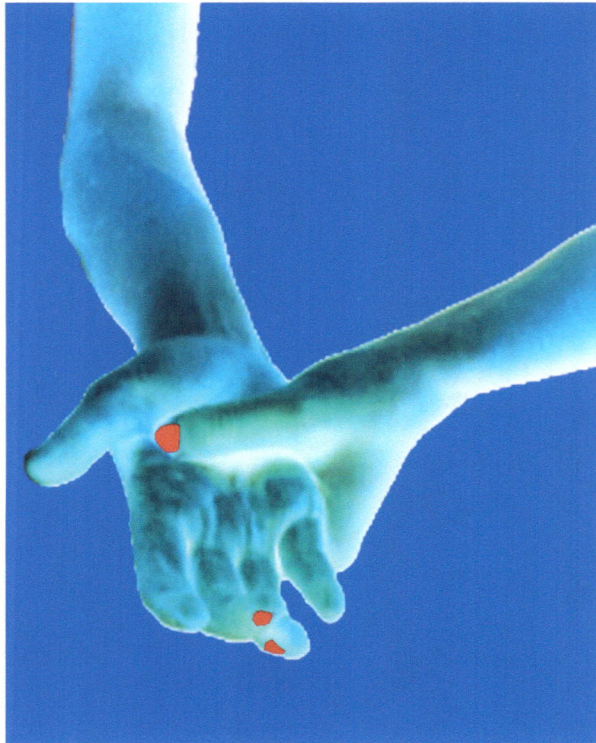

Picture 16. Self reflexology on the reflective area of the hand.

The reflective area at your hand, which is treated above with the thumb is connected to the stomach and digestive system. It is also entry point to the lung energy channel. The index finger below the thumb on the other side of the hand is pressing the entry point to the large intestine energy channel.

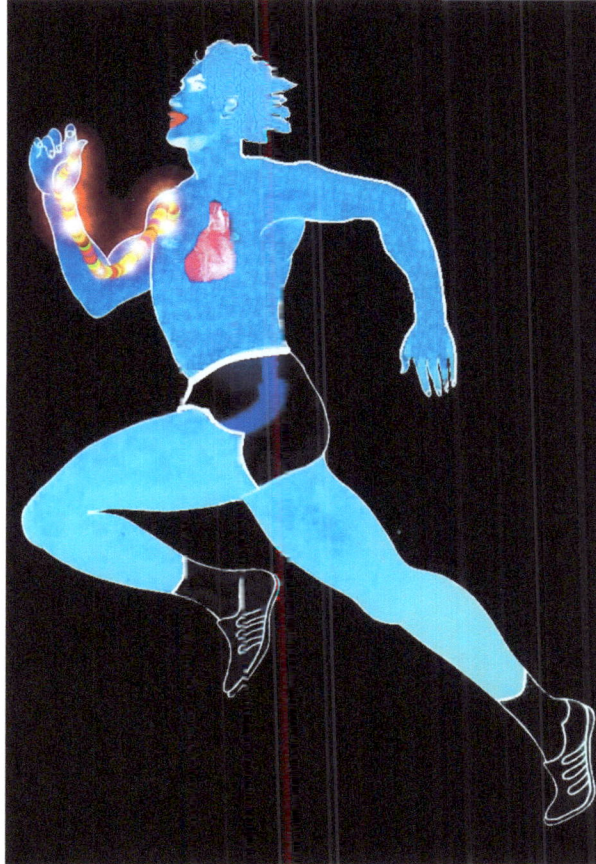

Picture 17. Lung energy channel.

The application and effect of the therapy are unique to each person. Your sensitive hands can detect imbalances, asymmetries, tiny deposits, tensions, micro-injuries of the ligaments, and much more. By working on these points, you can release the stagnation of vital energy flow.

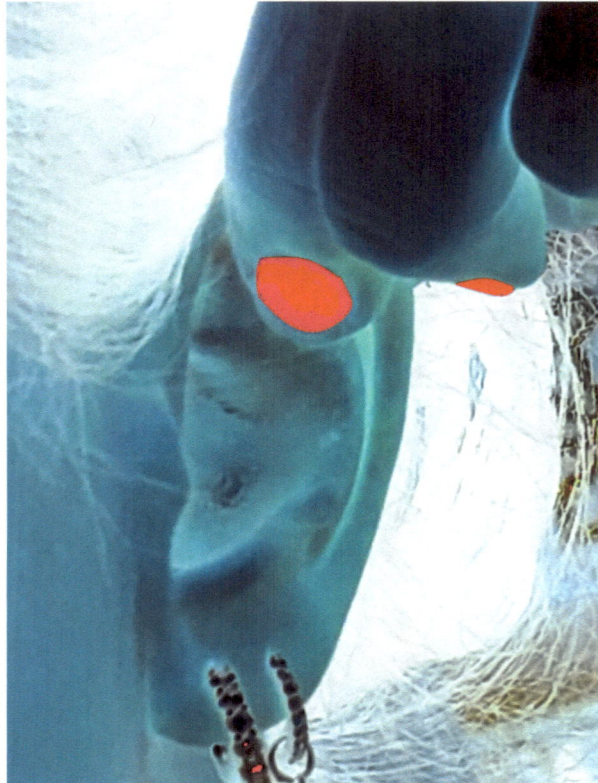

Picture 18. Ear reflexology.

Ear self-reflexology is easy to perform and safe. Pressure on the upper region of the ear has an anti-inflammatory effect. It needs to be exercised several times.

~ 6 ~

HAND REFLEXOLOGY

Hand reflexology, a time-honored art of applying the appropriate touch to the hands, can energize and restore health to other body parts, including internal organs. If you feel tired or have an infirmity, take a couple of minutes and just do it. This traditional medical approach to healing, deeply rooted in the wisdom of some Eastern and Western cultures, has been used for thousands of years.

Hand reflexology is the domain of using reflective areas on the hand. Reflexology explains how one part of the human body relates to another by applying mechanical impulses such as touch, pressure, and rubbing. Your hands contain many of the body's most potent reflective areas and are entry points to energy channels.

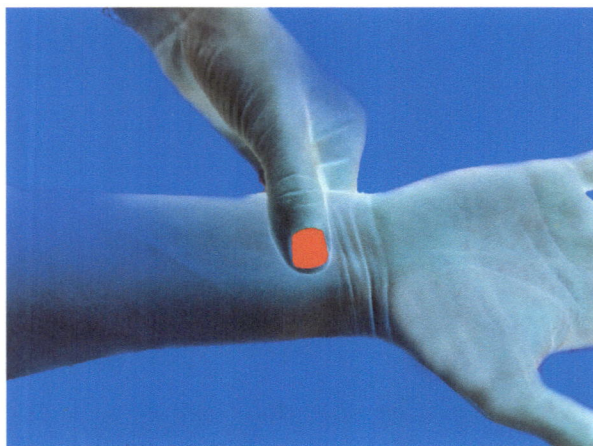

Picture 19. Reflective heart area. Courtesy Emerald.

It is easy to find and recognize the middle of the wrist. By applying gentle pressure to this area and rubbing with your thumb in a linear motion, you can relieve anxiety, insomnia, and heart palpitations. This area is sometimes referred to as the "inner gate" of the body. At the same time, it serves as the entry point for the pericardium energy channel, which is essential for lymphatic circulation. The pericardium is a sac containing a small amount of fluid that surrounds and protects the heart. This technique can be used by a therapist or for self-treatment.

The "outer gate" to your body is located on the opposite side of the wrist. To access both gates with one grip, press the entry point underneath the wrist with your thumb, while using your index finger to press at the outer gate. This area of outer gate to your body corresponds also to the triple energizer energy channel. To work on two reflective regions simultaneously, place two fingers from your other hand above your wrist—the thumb on the inner gate area and the index finger on the outer gate. Apply gentle pressure and either rub your fingers in circular motions or move them linearly over these sensitive areas. This technique can also be performed by a therapist or for self-treatment.

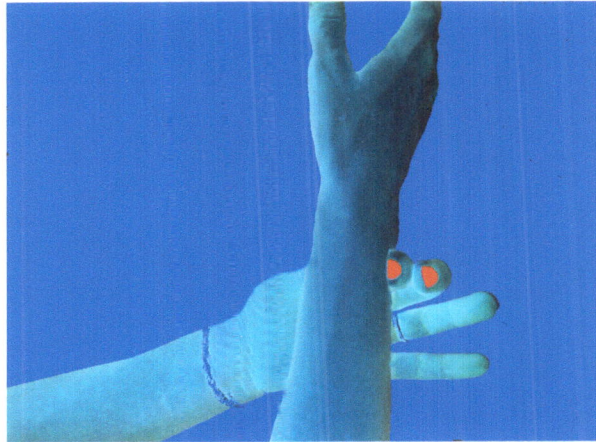

Picture 20. Reflective area for the inner and outer gate.
Courtesy Emerald.

Gently rubbing on both gates to your body with circular motions using your thumb and index finger can increase vital energy and sometimes it can result in a burst of an intense energy spreading instantly all over your body. Reflexology in this region enhance your immunity. It supports also stomach health and digestive function.

Another crucial reflective area for the improvement of the brain functionality and headaches can be found in the valley that forms when you stretch your thumb and index finger apart. The firm skin and connective tissue between these two fingers also serve as an entry point to the energy channel to the large intestine.

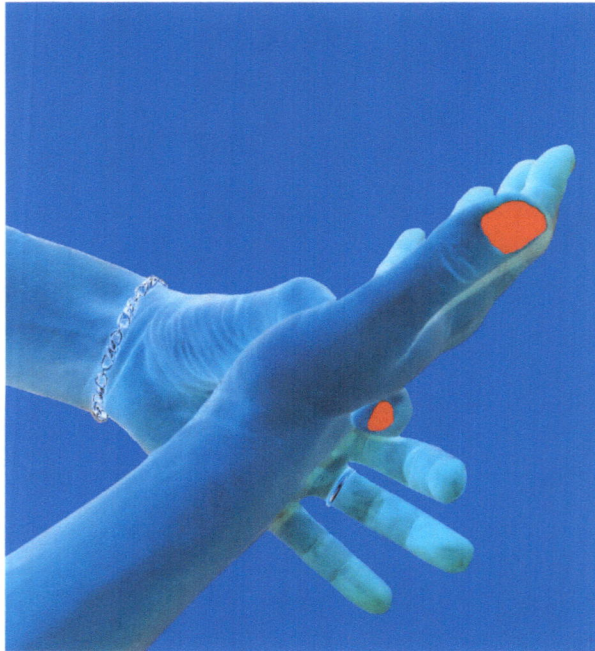

Picture 21. Reflective area for the head and brain.
Courtesy Emerald.

Applying firm pressure and using circular motions at the entry point of the large intestine energy channel is an effective technique for relieving stress and managing pain. This method can help to alleviate migraine, toothache, shoulder tension, and neck pain. It can be performed by a therapist or used for self-treatment, as illustrated in the accompanying picture.

Additionally, this technique can help reduce facial wrinkles, which often result from disturbed energy flow by incorrect chewing with the lower jaw and from existing infirmities in your digestive system. The energy channel of large intestine originates from the top of your index finger, then raises from this entry point between your thumb and index finger through the forearm, arm, shoulder, face, and upper lip, crossing over to the other side of the nose.

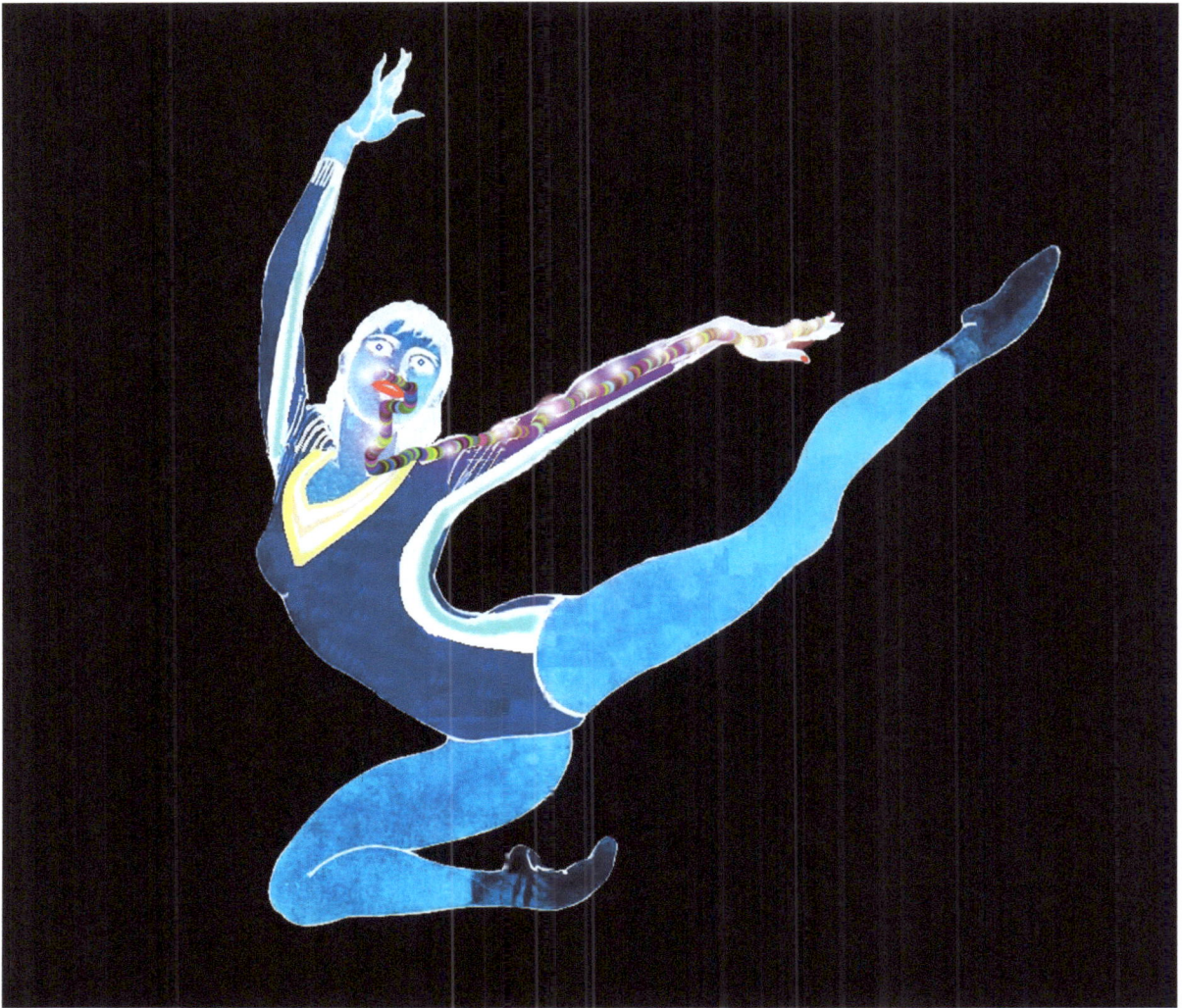

Picture 22. Large intestine energy channel.

The reflective area on the outer edge of your hand corresponds to the muscles of your neck and cervical spine. It is located in the depression below your small finger and contains the entry points for the small intestine energy channel. Applying firm pressure to this point helps to alleviate neck pain, shoulder tension, earaches, and headaches at the back of your head.

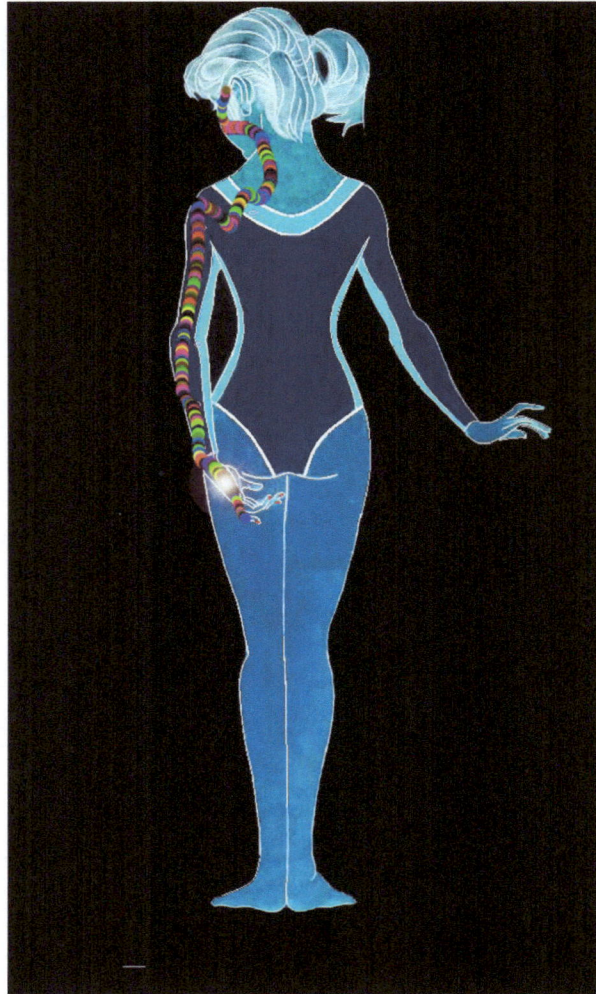

Picture 23. Small intestine energy channel. The reflective area outside of the edge of the hand is marked with light.

The next important reflective area on your hand at your palm along the edge of your thumb corresponds to your spine and spinal column.

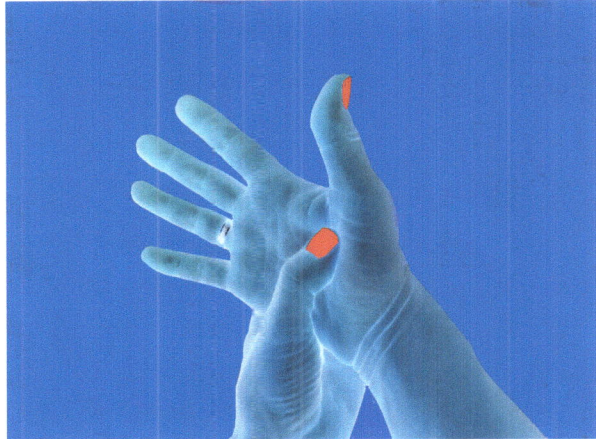

Picture 24. Reflective are for the spine on the thumb.
Courtesy Emerald.

The line, curved similarly to your spine, starts from the tip of your thumb and extends down the side of your hand, ending just beneath the crease of your wrist. Gently rub your thumb or fingers along this line, moving them up and down.

If you find any sore spots along the line, apply firm pressure and rub in small circles until the discomfort alleviates. You can use even your knuckles in this reflective area. This technique can help to manage lower back pain and may also terminate a persistent cough, as it connects to the entry points of your lung energy channel.

There is another clever grip in reflexology, which can boost your energy levels and strengthen your immune system. Applying pressure and rubbing the area between your thumb and index finger for the brain functions and the area for the spine and lungs functionality on the opposite side, at the same time, with two of your fingers stimulates two reflective areas and two important entry points can result in an intense rush of energy that spreads from your head to your toes throughout your body. Hand reflexology is a safe and proven method to enhance your health. Since it is non-invasive and does not involve pharmaceuticals, there is no risk of adverse side effects.

A trained reflexologist who has completed accredited training programs in reflexology or medical massage can provide secure and effective treatment, allowing you to explore this practical healing art confidently.

For sure you learn from your reflexologist how to stimulate your own reflective areas and energy channels at home. However, it is essential to educate yourself on the correct techniques to ensure safe and effective self-care.

While reflexology is a traditional form of medicine, it can complement your existing medical treatments. It should not replace visits to your medical doctor or general practitioner, but it can enhance your recovery process and support your overall health, providing a holistic approach to well-being. Experts affirm that reflexology is unlikely to cause any adverse effects on the body, making it entirely safe for practice. Its non-invasive nature and accessibility make it a highly inclusive and effective therapeutic aid, available to anyone seeking its benefits.

~ 7 ~

TALE OF KIDS' REFLEXOLOGY

In a faraway land, there is a serene billabong where a deer with its imposing antlers approaches crystal clear water, and a white wild cat gracefully navigates its own way through the blossoming bush in spring a pretty Queen and a strong, noble King had their palace.

In this land, where the sea mirrors the azure tones of the summer sky and reflects the warm sun, where in autumn in the countryside. white pelican dances with a vibrant rainbow, the Queen and the King fell in love in this marvelous and enchanting land. In this ferry-tale land where kangaroos stand around and listen and look for mangoes, admiring the beauty of the Christmas trees, a beautiful boy is looking from heaven to find the right parents.

The Queen and the King were known as light adorers because their most admired colors were the sun's white and yellow. They were deeply in love, and their passion for each other was soon blessed with an exceptional child who would lead a new generation of young people in their kingdom.

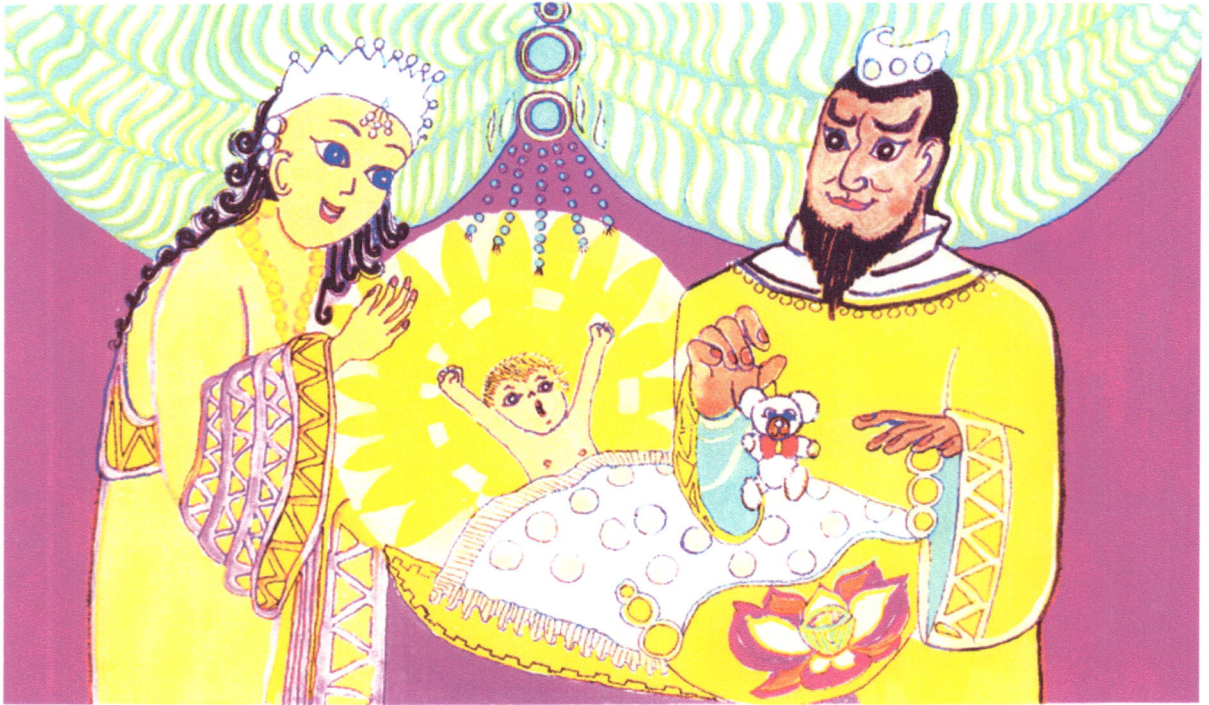

Picture 25. Queen and King received the boy. Courtesy Angela Rudhart-Dyczynski.

The newborn child was lovely and good-looking, with deep, dark, sparkling eyes full of light. He had strong, glossy hair. The King and Queen were proud of his soft, bright skin and dressed their kid in fine linen and beautiful, colorful fabrics.

His room was marvelous, adorned with artistic furniture. Through the big window, playful sunshine surrounded his crawling and the first unsteady steps on the soft rugs. The kid grew up in this space, each day a new adventure, in peace, with the love of the Queen and King always creating a cheerful atmosphere around him. His life was full of sweet fragrances, the finest food, and beautiful toys.

This is a marvelous world, thought the kid more often. This is the world I have been promised in the tummy of the Queen, and I have waited for so long. The vital breath murmured in its lungs, and its sweetheart pounded when it faced the strong and meaningful life impressions.

The kid smiled, looked around him with the utmost interest, played with its tiny hands and feet, and shouted, sometimes loud and bold while enjoying the beautiful movements of his chest caused by his vital breath. It wanted to repeat the breath movement again and again.

He then slept, tired and overjoyed from the world's impressions and intense experiences.

The time passed quickly, and after days, weeks, and months, the kid grew stronger and stronger.

Unexpected came an illness upon the beautiful kid of the Queen and King, and its eventful and bright life became cold and dark. He cried and shouted loudly day and night without end. His eyes lost the sparks and stopped reflecting the light. His greasy hair was not shiny, and his pale face contrasted with the dark on the white cushion in the background of the colorful bed. The kid looked as weak and infirm.

The palace doctor was called in but could not help the child. The King and the Queen sent messengers all over the Sunshine Kingdom to look after a natural healer who could heal their ill child.

One day, a wise man in a long, deep blue mantle knocked at the palace door. He was an experienced healer and had healed many kids in his peaceful and charitable life. He understood the healing and secret of heaven. He also was skilled in martial arts and knew the healing power of nature and Earth. His and Her Excellencies have summoned me, so I am here. Please place the kid in a cozy bed on a large, soft towel and bring me a fragrant mineral oil, he instructed, setting the scene for the healing to come.

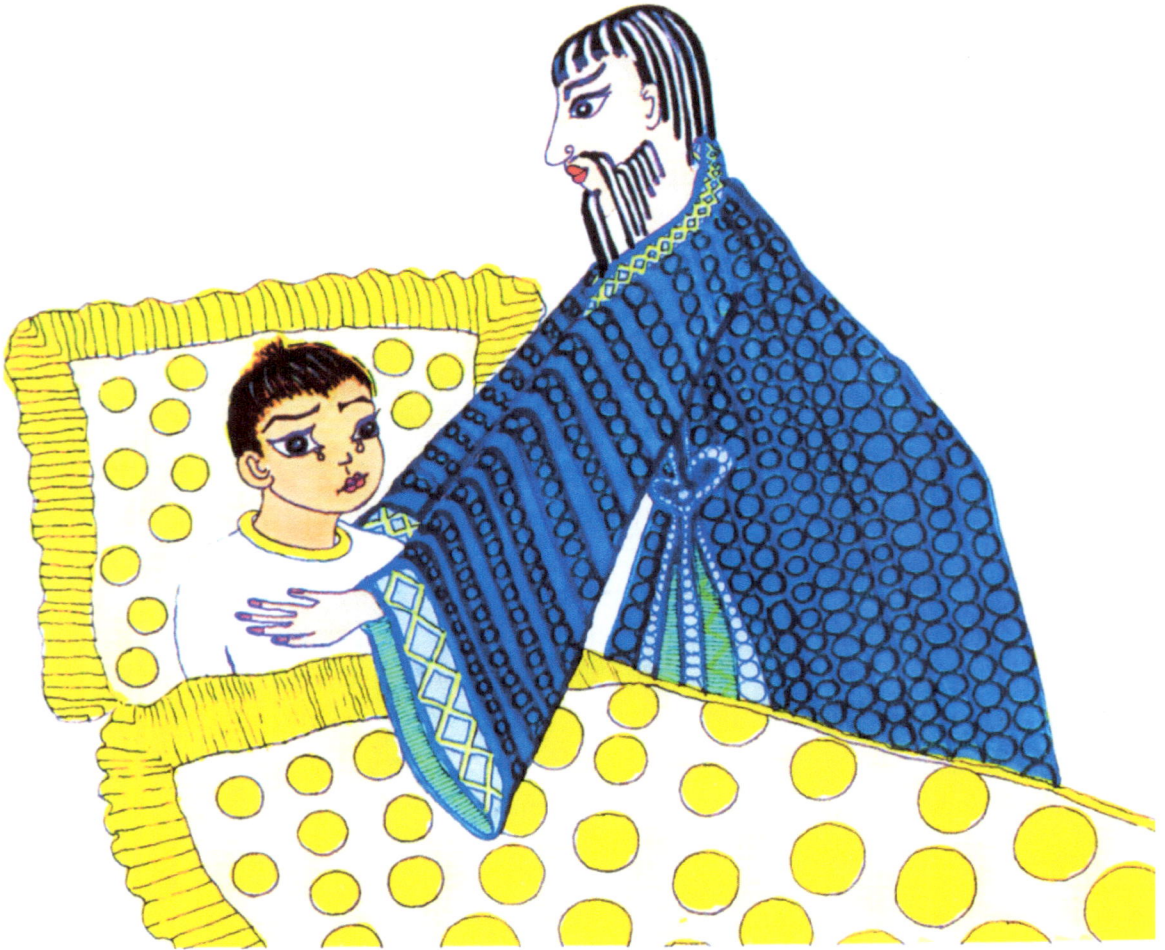

Picture 26. The Healer treating the boy. Courtesy Angela Rudhart-Dyczynski.

The Queen and the King did according to the wise man's advice. The experienced Healer looked at him with empathy. You are a handsome and beautiful kid, he spoke to it. He took the small hand in his strong palm and said, "You will be healthy soon, smiling, dancing, jumping, and singing as long as you want." He quickly moved his hand as frequently as he spoke, gently rubbing and pressing the kid's hands and arms, focusing on specific places on the palm and fingers. His skillful fingers accelerated the movements, becoming almost indistinct, but the kid liked it more and more. Then, he put his fingers in a small bowl filled with fragrant and natural oil and moved his hand alongside the kid's fingers, arms, and shoulders.

To the King and Queen, observing the Healer, it seemed as if their son was receiving invisible life impulses from the Healer's hands. Their kid stopped crying, and his eyes regained their light. He watched with interest as the Healer changed the locations between his hands, arms, shoulders, and head and became receptive and curious about the healing happening to his now strengthened body.

The King and Queen were amazed at the transformation their infirm kid experienced after being treated by the wise Healer. After being wrapped in a cozy towel, he fell asleep with a rosy complexion and deep relaxation. They asked the Healer, "How did you do it?"

The wise Healer replied. I will be honest with you. The potential for complete healing is always present. It can be awakened by the right stimulus, such as the touch of your hands and the energy they carry when applied to the kid's skin, muscles, and tendons. The healing power of your hands can surpass that of fire, water, trees, and even the strongest metals.

The key is to synchronize the frequency of your hand movements with the child's heartbeat, which is much faster than that of adults, whose hearts usually beat 60 to 70 times per minute.

Please remember what I am now saying to you, Your Majesty, and my Queen. Your frequency of hand movements has to be at least twice as quick as the adults, and then the kid can take it in with its whole body. The kid's body vibrates according to its frequent heartbeats, about 120 to 160 in a minute. The younger the kid, the more frequent the heartbeat. The baby's and infants' fast heartbeat frequency is even higher, up to 180 beats per minute. Your kid is a couple of years old, so you must move your fingers and hands about 120 times a minute. You can use a little oil as it allows the kid's body to discharge abnormal electromagnetic potential. The minerals contained in this oil accelerate the energy flow. Your hand's rubbing moves will relax the tense muscles, making the body field more stable.

The greatest secret for healing lies in your kid's hands. I will tell you about the secrets of kid's fingers. The middle finger is the King, which relates to the heart, the body's central organ. The fourth finger is the Queen, which represents the lungs. If you rub each finger with gentle pressing and small circular moves, it will strengthen the heart and the lungs. This invisible healing energy of your parental hands can be a thousand times more potent than any other medicine applied to a kid for healing. If you practice diligently, you will discover that your hands are the healing hands.

I will equip you with the necessary knowledge and train you in this art of healing for your kid. On this day, the wise Healer stayed in the palace until late at night and gave his knowledge about the way they need to act as the parents and the doctors alike so that the illness can be cured.

You need to rub the kid's fingers with gentle, quick movements. You massage his hands first. The fingers are the most essential parts.

The middle finger, the King, is connected to the heart, and the fourth finger is the Queen as it relates to the child's lungs. During the massage of these fingers, the intelligent functions of the heart and lungs will be strengthened. The lungs and the heart generally govern the fundamental aspects of the Kingdom of the kid's body. The second finger is the General, which represents the liver and gallbladder. The thumb is the representation of the stomach and spleen. I call it the Minister for the Kingdom's supply, as the power resulting from food digestion is transformed into a great strength of the immune system. The fifth, last, and smallest finger is the Healer, representing the genetics, kidney system, and adrenals with their greatest potential to support healing.

There is a sea of vital energy in the middle of the hand. You need to circle with your fingers around and in the middle of this energy ocean. This sea is connected directly to the heart's healing power and the brain, which oversees the intelligent healing processes.

The next day, the Queen and the King began treating their kid with their own hands, and his skin became softer and healthier. He grew stronger over the following weeks and months, and his posture became more solid. They noticed that his intelligence developed in enormous leaps. He enjoyed his daily reflexology. Due to their duties in the Sunshine Kingdom, the Queen and the King sometimes missed giving their beloved child a gentle reflexology for a day. On those occasions, their child was not really happy.

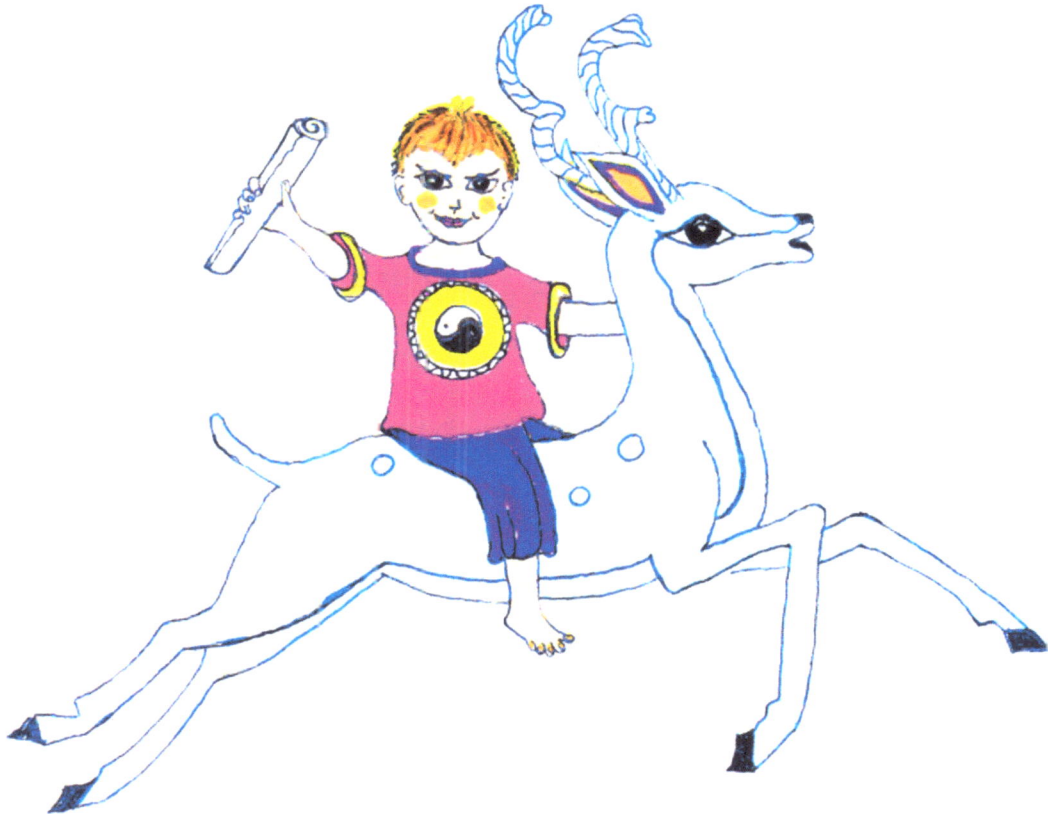

Picture 27. The healed kid riding on the deer. Courtesy Angela Rudhart-Dyczynski.

The King and Queen of the Sunshine Kingdom were committed to ensuring the health and wellness of all kids. They understood the importance of the reflexology techniques. They documented the knowledge of the wise Healer as high-priority health advice. Their commitment to sharing this knowledge throughout the entire Kingdom was unwavering.

~ 8 ~

KIDS REFLEXOLOGY

*L*et the little children come to me, and do not hinder them, for the kingdom of God belongs to such
*as these. Truly I tell you, anyone who will not receive the kingdom of God like a little child will
never enter it." And he took the children in his arms, placed his hands on them and blessed them.
Matthew Chapter19. Verse 14-15.*

The soothing, gentle reflexology for kids has a long-standing value in traditional medicine. The kid's reflexology technique is an excellent practice that helps promote the healing and development of kids, both physically and intellectually. The authors studied this technique in 1991 and 1992 at the Beijing Massage Hospital in China, specifically at the Pediatric Department for Kids.

During this time, the hospital primarily used massage, reflexology, and herbal teas as therapeutic approaches for adults and children. Witnessing kids being treated for bronchitis, pneumonia, gastrointestinal, and neurological disorders with reflexology and herbs led the authors to question whether reflexology and natural medicine can treat the majority of childhood infirmities.

From today's perspective, our answer is clear, consistent, and accurate: The kids must benefit from a combination of traditional and modern medicine, ensuring safety and effectiveness in any therapeutic approach.

Our children deserve more than what the modern world offers, such as big screen TVs, smartphones, artificial intelligence, and overloaded school curricula focusing on early learning. They need genuine love from their parents. As parents, it is your responsibility to provide this emotional connection through touch, physical communication, hugs, dedication, and quality time together. Without this connection, children may be labeled as overactive or might retreat into their own world, isolating themselves from the emotional support they need.

The energy pathways differ a bit between kids and adults; however, there is solid and common ground to consider the energy channels similarly, knowing that kids' channels are constantly developing. In contrast, adults' channels are mature and have less plasticity.

The kid's energy pathways are broader and cover with their streams kids' bodies, much like the rivers on the Earth in the wet season. Kids' muscle and skin pathways are undifferentiated, developing into full-functioning energy channels over time. The body of a kid is more transparent and integrated in the nature.

It takes about 10 to 12 years for the energy channels to fully develop and mature in their functionality, a process completed with puberty.

Kids' reflexology is a technique that is adaptable to their age and developmental state, ensuring safety and effectiveness.

For instance, a baby's reflexology focuses primarily on the fingers, hands, and underarms. Reflexology for a kid approaching puberty will concentrate on the muscle pathways in the hands, arms, spine, and feet. This adaptability of reflexology treatment to the kid's age reassures parents about the safety and effectiveness of the applied reflexology, ensuring their child's unique needs are being met.

From birth, babies and young kids explore the world primarily using their hands as their general senses are not fully developed. This is why the hand as a target for healing intervention is predominantly essential.

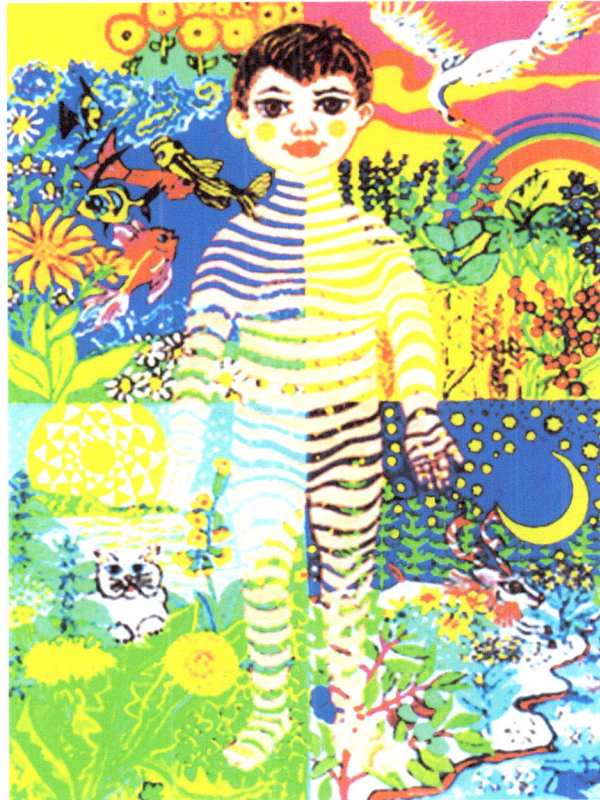

Picture 28. A kid's body with nature and four seasons.

Courtesy Angela Rudhart -Dyczynski.

Kid's energy channels do not have distinct entry points; they have larger areas with more blood vessels, receptors, and collagen fibers. Over time, these areas condense and develop into energy channels with specific entry points.

Reflexology performed by parents not only relaxes their kids but also triggers the release of beneficial hormones, activates the immune system, and accelerates detoxification. This holistic approach to healing through reflexology instills a sense of hope and positive feelings in parents, who know that they are holistically contributing to their kid's health and comprehensively promoting their development and well-being.

~ 9 ~

PARENTS GUIDE TO KIDS REFLEXOLOGY

The gentle kid's reflexology can have a particular sequence to reach the full healing potential. Parents play a crucial role in creating a suitable environment for reflexology.

Finding a quiet, secure space and creating a warm and inviting atmosphere is essential. If the room is too cold, you can use a red or heat lamp to help maintain the proper temperature, showing dedication to your kid's comfort. Use a fresh, large, soft towel to cover the area where your kid will lie, whether on a bed or a treating table.

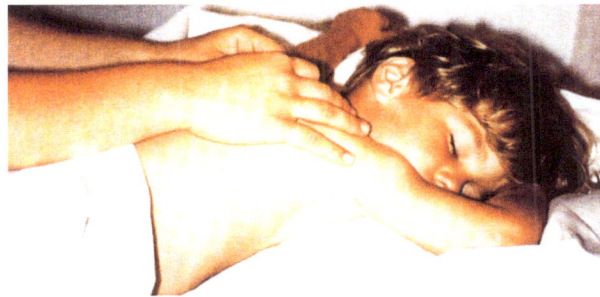

Picture 29. Relaxed kid after reflexology.

Safety is paramount. For a safe and gentle experience, use baby oil to rub your fingers, and consider using either Arnica oil or other suitable oils that your child tolerates well. After the gentle kids' reflexology, your kid will need to rest.

Remember, the post-reflexology time is as important as the gentle intervention itself. This time enables the kid's body to fully absorb the benefits of the reflexology, giving you peace of mind that you are doing everything possible for your kid's health. Ensuring your kid gets the most out of the reflexology treatment is crucial.

As you begin the reflexology treatment, remember that you are not just a parent but also a therapist. Starting with the kid's left hand is a strategic move. It helps establish a connection with the right part of the brain, as the nerves from the left part of the body cross in the cervical spine to the right hemisphere of the brain.

Gentle kid's reflexology is a comprehensive treatment that consists of two parts. The first part includes reflexology on the hands, fingers, and forearms. The second part consists of longer rubbing moves of the muscle pathways, running alongside the arms, chest, legs, feet, and spine.

~ 10 ~

KID'S HAND REFLEXOLOGY

The hand, palm, and fingers of your kid are the ultimate gateways for healing. The first grip of your hand should target the area at the kid's left wrist, as shown in the image below. Your index finger on the left hand should be the support, while your thumb on the right should be the reflexology tool.

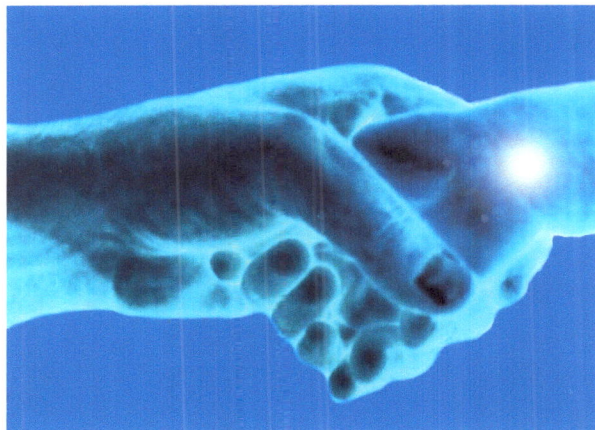

Picture 30. Essential grip of kid's hand reflexology.

The illustration of the fundamental, essential grip for the kid's reflexology of the hand provides a visual guide to help you understand the correct hand positioning and pressure application. Hold the kid's hand firmly and apply a small amount of pressure. Gently tilt the wrist so that the area of interest moves towards your thumb. With your thumb, make a circular rubbing movement.

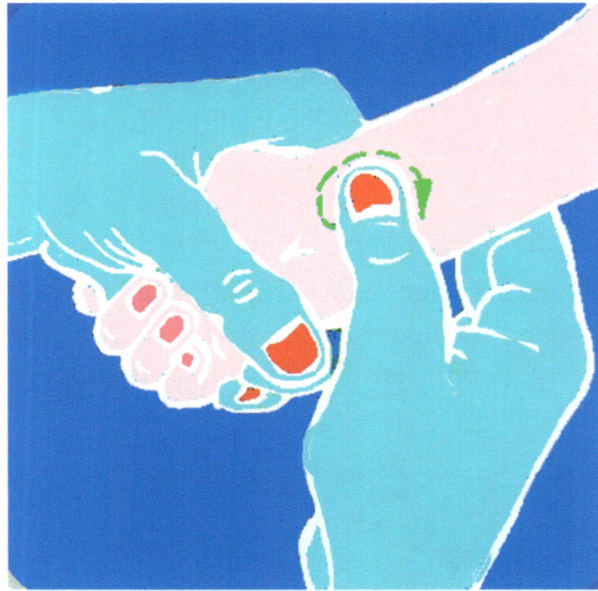

Picture 31. Circular rubbing using essential grip.
Courtesy Angela Rudhart-Dyczynski.

The circular massage of an area at the wrist to connect emotionally with the kid. The movement frequency should be similar to a kid's heartbeat, which is faster than an adult's, typically between 100 and 120 movements per minute. If you want to energize your kid, move your hand more frequently.

Each finger of your kid needs your attention. Remember, the hand is the ultimate gateway to your kid's health. Your care and attention can make a significant difference. Remember you guide your kid to well-feeling and well-being.

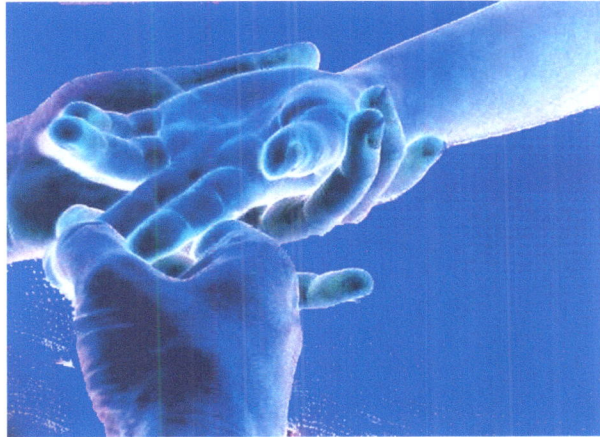

Picture 32. The reflexology of the fingers.

The reflexology technique for the fingers and fingertips, like the wrist, is simple and easy to perform. Two fingers are active, with the thumb rubbing linearly or circularly. Simultaneously, the fingertip of the index finger provides counter pressure and buffers the movements, making it straightforward.

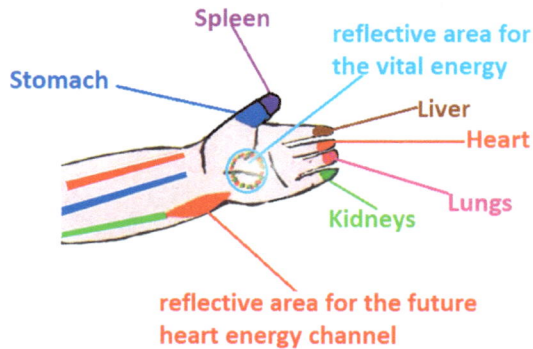

Picture 33. The reflective areas at the fingers and the lines on the forearm.

The reflective areas on your kid's fingers correspond to various internal organs and body parts. By gently rubbing or pressing these areas for about 30 seconds, you can stimulate the nerve endings in the fingers, which may positively impact the connected organs or body parts.

When starting a reflexology session, it is essential to begin with your kid's middle finger, often referred to as the King. This finger is significantly linked to the heart, one of the most vital organs in the body.

Next, focus on the fourth finger, known as the Queen', which is associated with the lungs. Understanding these connections empowers you as a parent to support your kid's health effectively.

While performing reflexology, it is also important to pay attention to your kid's breathing. Typically, kids breath starts in the belly region. You can observe the diaphragm's movement around kid's belly button. However, the breathing of your kid can sometimes default to upper chest and shoulder breathing, which is less effective.

Encouraging correct breathing can positively influence your kid's health and well-being. One fun way to achieve this is to start a friendly competition to see who can take more belly breaths—either you or your kid. This activity often leads to laughter and helps release tension in you and in your kid's body.

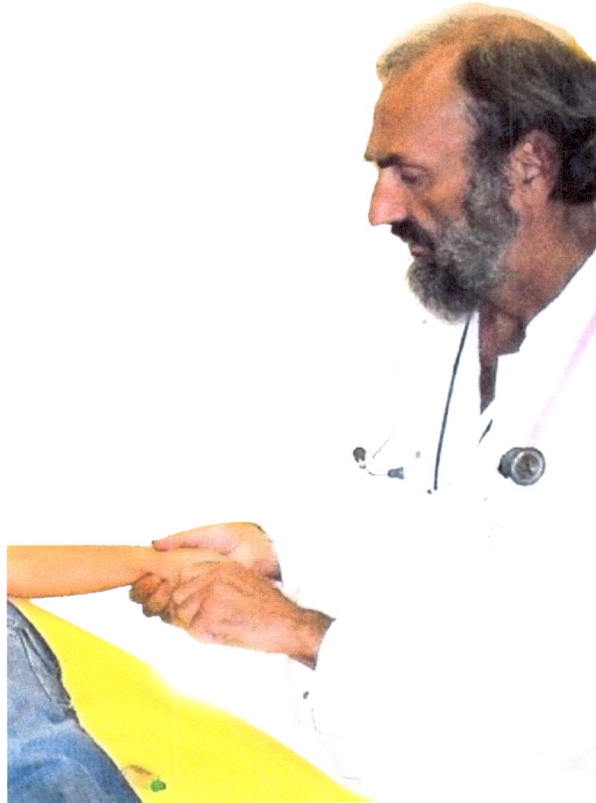

Picture 34. Dr. George makes reflexology on the kid's fingers.

Your role in your kid's reflexology is most important. By focusing entirely on reflective areas, you actively contribute to your kid's health and well-being, strengthening you as a parent.

The index finger, represents the liver and gallbladder. This area balances the kid's energy production, and your stimulation on this reflective area counteracts its stress reactions.

The thumb is a reflective connection to the spleen and stomach, both organs contributing to its natural and effective digestive functions.

The small fifth finger is a reflective connection to the kid's kidneys and adrenals. This finger is known as a healer in reflexology because it relates to the genetics of your kid and the enormous healing potential that can be released from the adrenals, especially Cortisol, with its anti-inflammatory features.

Please remember reflexology is adaptable. Rub the corresponding areas more frequently depending on your kid's symptoms. For example, during reflexology treatment, if your kid is experiencing bloating, belly pain, or diarrhea, focus on the thumb, index finger, and small finger. Your adaptability to the kid's needs, based on careful observation of its behavior and reaction to the applied impulses, gives you confidence in managing your kid's health with excellence.

Reflexology is a powerful tool for managing your kid's mood and health. There are many reflective areas on the back of the forehand, back of the hand, and fingers. These areas relate to the function of your kid's internal organs including the heart and brain. If you would influence your kids' over-reactivity or improve her/his altered mood, please focus on the top of the fingers just above the nails and joints. These areas have reflective connections to your kid's brain. You can use reflexology in these areas when you would like to calm your overexcited kid. They are marked as blue circles with white spots.

.

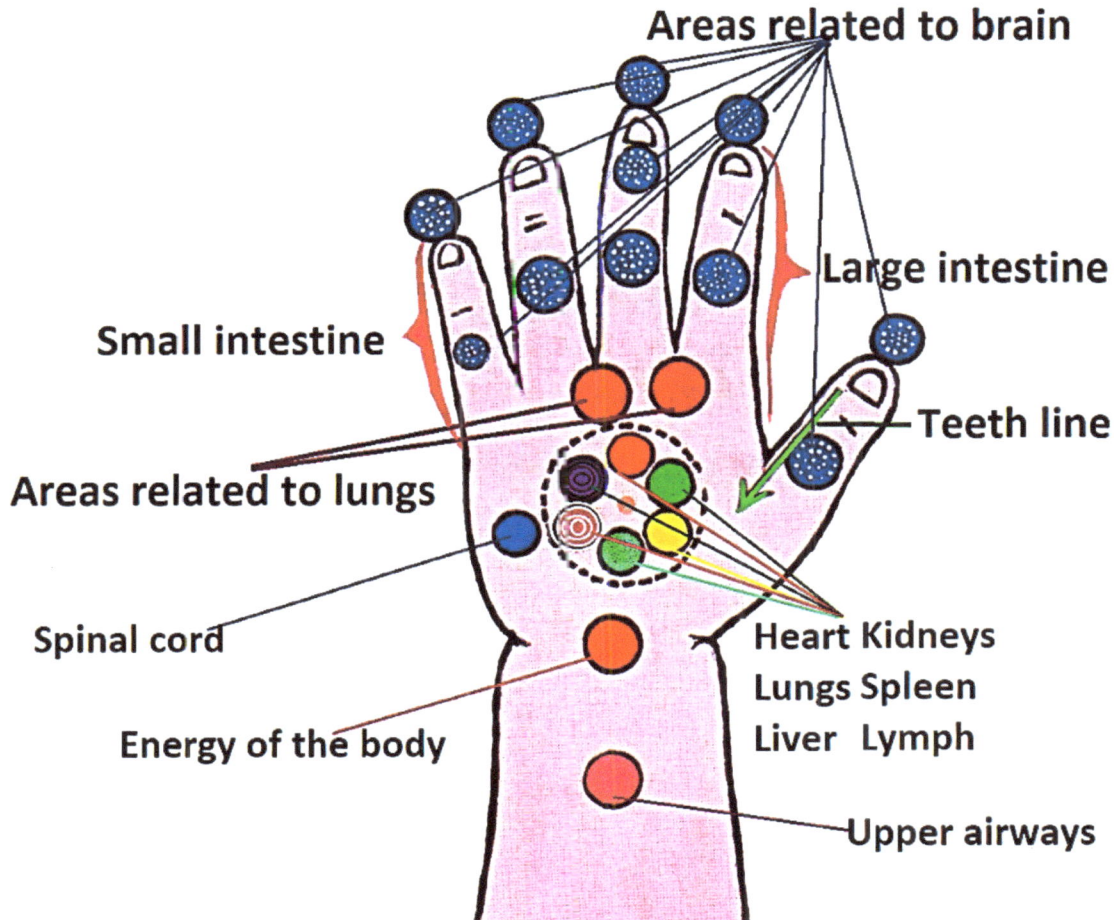

Picture 35. Reflexology on the back of the forehand, hand and fingers.

A line marked with a green arrow has a reflective connection to your kid's face and teeth. The round, deep red spots highlight areas linked to the lungs and upper airways. This reflexology map on the back of your kid's hand is a valuable guide to understanding organ connections.

The area that corresponds to the small intestine is located on the outer surface of the little finger, while the area related to the large intestine is found on the outer surface of the index finger. Gently rubbing along this line can help alleviate bloating, abdominal colic, or gas pain caused by indigestion.

One of the most beneficial reflexology techniques is the circular, rubbing in circles moves on the back of the kid's hand. These moves deliver reflective impulses and improve the function of the most essential internal organs: heart, lung, liver, kidneys, spleen, and pericardium, a part of the lymphatic system.

By rubbing this area with the circular movement of the thumb or two fingers, you can significantly enhance your kid's health. The area over the wrist marked with red relates to your kid's bodily energy production and metabolism. The area marked with a deep blue color at the outer side of the backhand refers to the spinal cord and brain functionality.

Inclusion of these reflective areas in your reflexology can promote a happier, healthier kid!

~ 11 ~

REFLEXOLOGY OF THE KIDS FOREARMS

After finishing the treatment for the kid's hands, the next step is to concentrate on performing linear, quick movements along the three lines in the forearm. Begin with the blue balancing line in the middle, then move to the green line associated with the internal organs, and finally, address the red vitality line.

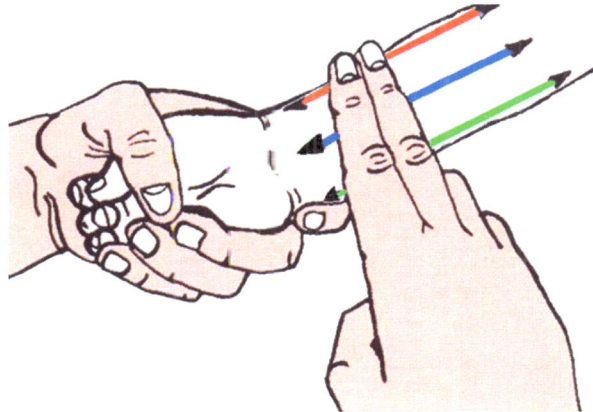

Picture 36. Reflexology on three lines of the forearm.
Courtesy Angela Rudhart-Dyczynski.

It s important to remember that your kid is your teacher, and you should adjust your reflexology techniques according to his/her reactions. While you are the parent, you also need to act as a therapist and an knowledgeable observer, please pay close attention to the signs and symptoms while performing reflexology on your kid. Signs refer to what you observe visually, while symptoms relate to your kid's reactions and feelings that you notice.

Begin the reflexology by focusing on the blue line on the forearm, which corresponds to the heart functions. Use two fingers to gently rub this line up and down. Observe your kid carefully during this process. Once you feel satisfied with the sensations and responses of your kid, switch to the other parallel line.

Effective reflexology will lead to a pinkish-red color appearing on the skin of the forearms. Working on the red line helps boost your kid's vitality. This line is linked to the heart, brain, and emotions. Your high frequent rubbing will work to balance and calm kid's body.

The green line represents your kid's internal transport organs and is very important for reflexology. It is connected to the organs that transport food, nutrients, and bodily fluids, including the stomach, small intestine, large intestine, urinary bladder, gall bladder, and the pericardium at the core of the lymphatic system. Understanding these connections will optimize your technique and guide your fingers during the reflexology session.

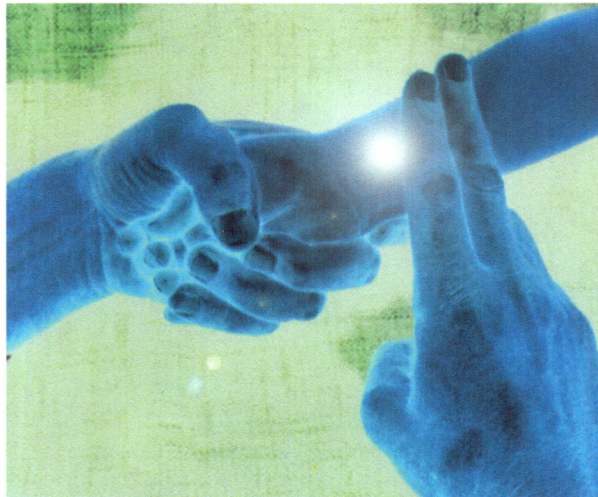

Picture 37. Reflexology on the balancing line in the middle.

After an invigorating reflexology with your focus on the three lines at the forearm, it is paramount to help your kids to enhance their lung function. You can do it by gently rubbing the area beneath the collarbone with two fingers, which contributes to the normalization of your kid's sensibility.

This reflexology technique is effective in resetting the breathing to its optimal functionality. To begin, use two fingers to make linear movements at a quick frequency of about 100 movements per minute. It is important to be careful and attentive during this process, as this area is sensitive. If your kid appears uncomfortable or unhappy with your reflexology technique, switch to the other side or return to the lines on the forearms or the tips of your kid's fingers.

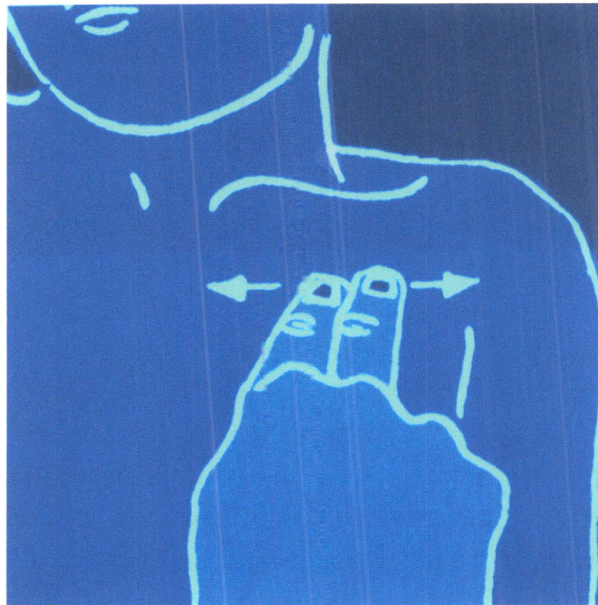

Picture 38. Invigorating the function of the lungs.

Reflexology is a powerful tool for managing your kid's mood and emotional health. There are many reflective areas on the back of the forehand, back of the hand, and fingers. These areas relate to the function of your kid's internal organs. If you would like to influence your kids' over-reactivity or her/his mood swings, please focus on the top of the fingers just above the nails and joints. These areas have reflective connections to your kid's brain and can calm imbalances in brain chemicals.

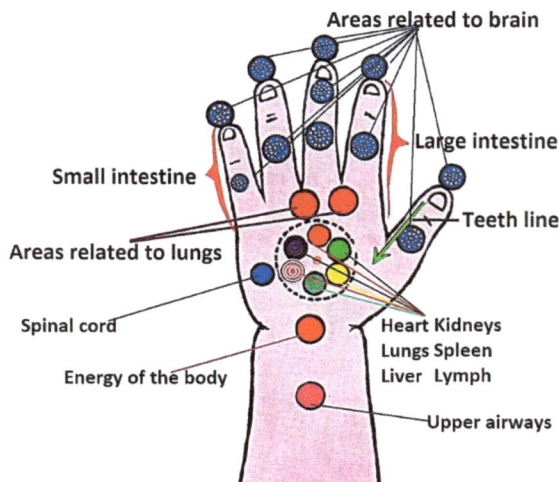

Picture 39. Reflective areas on the back of the kid's hand.

You can use reflexology in these areas when you would like to calm your distressed or overexcited kid. To help you identify these areas, they are marked with blue circles with white spots, which indicate their significance in reflexology.

There is a line marked with a green arrow, which has a reflective connection to your kid's teeth. This line is significant in reflexology as it guides you to the areas related to the lungs and upper airways, which are marked with burgundy color. The area with a reflective relation to the small intestine is at the outer surface of the small finger and at the outer surface of the index finger to the large intestine. The linear rubbing of this line is helpful for bloating, abdominal colic, or tummy pain caused by indigestion.

One of the most beneficial reflexology techniques is the circular, big rubbing moves on the back of the kid's hand. These moves deliver reflective impulses and improve the function of the most essential internal organs: heart, lung, liver, kidneys, spleen, and pericardium, a part of the lymphatic system. You can significantly enhance your kid's health by rubbing this area with the circular movement of the thumb or two fingers. The area over the wrist marked with red relates to your kid's bodily energy production and metabolism. The area marked with a deep blue color at the outer side of the backhand is the reflective part of the hand, which refers to the spinal cord.

These visual cues on the reflexology map on the backhand of the kid are significant as they guide you to the areas with reflective connections to specific organs.

~ 12 ~

LONG MOVES OF REFLEXOLOGY

Gentle reflexology can also be beneficial for your kid's muscle pathways. The spine and the spinal cord play a leading role in your kid's ongoing development and require special attention. The spinal cord supplies nerves to all muscles, internal organs, and the skin. These nerves branch out from the spinal cord, connecting with both the skin and muscles. As shown in the image below, there are many important reflex areas on a kid's back.

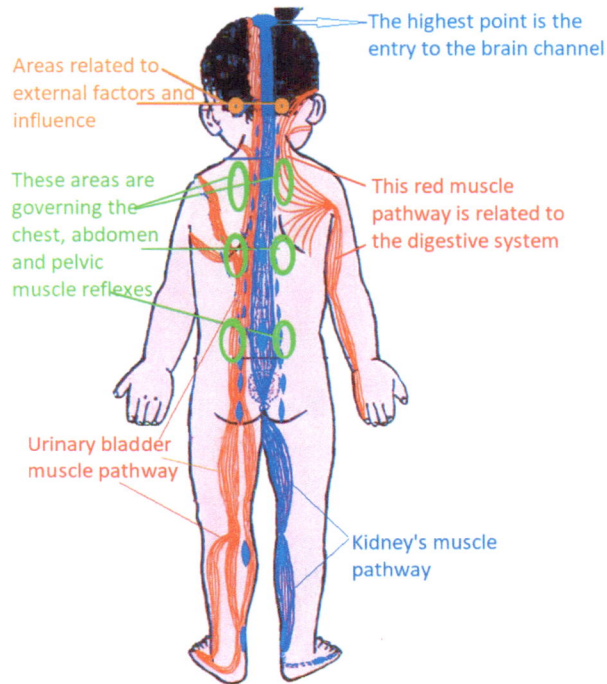

Picture 40. The long muscle pathways and reflective areas on kid's back.

Long reflexology moves will be performed on the muscles beside the spine. The gentle pressure of your thumbs will stimulate the dynamic spinal response resulting in wave like muscle moves in the green-marked areas.

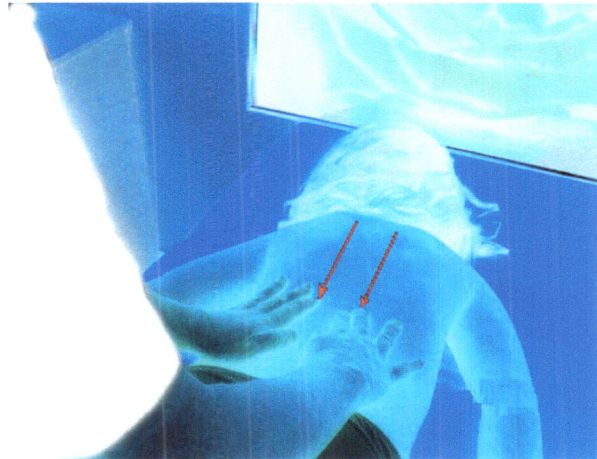

Picture 41. Illustration of the long moves reflexology on the back of a kid.

This visual guide will help you identify the key areas to focus on during a reflexology session. To perform back reflexology, begin with long moves along the muscle pathways on either side of the spine, moving from the neck down to the lower back. Use the pressure of your index and middle finger and apply a firm touch as you move close to the spine.

YOUR SEQUENCE OF KID'S REFLEXOLOGY

The order of your individualized kid reflexology.

Eight steps guide.

1.Establishment of the emotional connection.
The essential grip at the wrist and circular movements at the inside of the wrist establish an emotional connection with your kid. Remember to tilt your kid's wrist slightly and adjust the circular rubbing to your kid's age. The younger your kid is, the more frequently you move your thumb.

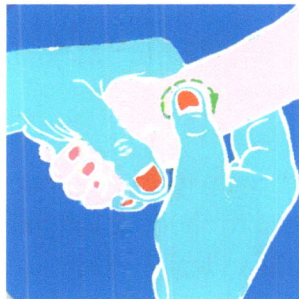

Picture 43. The essential grip with circular rubbing.

2. Energizing your kid's body.

Perform reflexology on the three lines of the forearm starting with the middle line. Please treat every line for at least 30 seconds. The efficiency of your moves will be seen in the rose color of the rubbed skin.

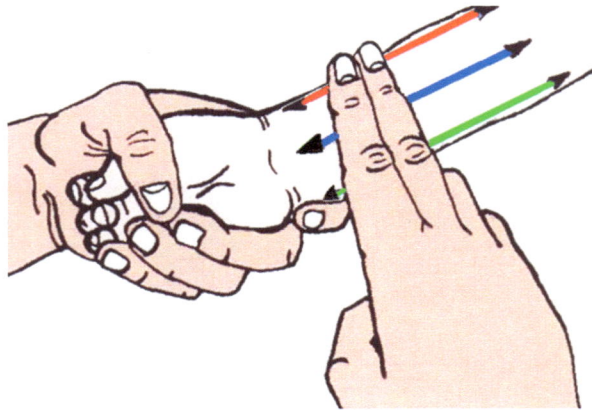

Picture 43. Reflexology on three lines of the forearm.

3. Royal treatment of the fingers.

Reflexology of the fingers begins with the left hand, followed by the right hand. It is important to follow this recommended order:

- The King (the heart) - please start with the middle finger.
- The Queen (the lungs) - proceed to the ring finger.
- The General (the liver and gallbladder) - is the index finger.
- The Minister of Supply (the thumb).
- The Healer (the kidneys and adrenals, known for their healing potential) - finish with the small finger.

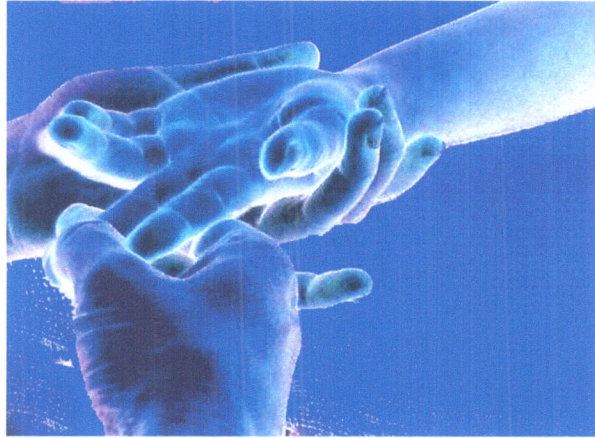

Picture 44. Reflexology on the fingers.

By following this sequence, you can effectively engage in reflexology for both hands of your kid.

4. Boosting of immunity, energy and blood supply.

The reflexology on the wrist and thumb reflective areas will lift up the energy production and the blood supply to the internal organs. Perform the reflexology of the fingertips focusing on the third finger longer, as it is representing the reflective area of the heart. It will increase the blood supply to the whole body of your kid. If you perform it correctly your kid's complexion of the face skin will become more natural, sparkling in texture and it will appear in more rose color.

Then switch to the fingertip of the fourth finger, as it relates in a reflective way to your kid's lungs. Remember that infections of the upper airways and lungs are widespread in childhood.

You can continue with the reflexology of the two areas of the thumb, the tip which relates to the stomach, marked with blue, and the lower part of the thumb which is the reflective area for the spleen marked with violet color. This is the boost for the immune system of your kid. The fifth fingertip needs also your longer attention because the kidneys and adrenals play critical roles in healing. The red area will be vital for your kid's heart energy channel in the future, so it is good to support this region with an energetic linear move using two-finger rubbing in a frequent linear way.

At the end you can focus on the index finger and perform reflexology there, remembering that it relates to the liver and gallbladder, symbolically known in traditional medicine as the General. It has a calming effect as the gallbladder is in charge of the hormones production involved in emotional reactions.

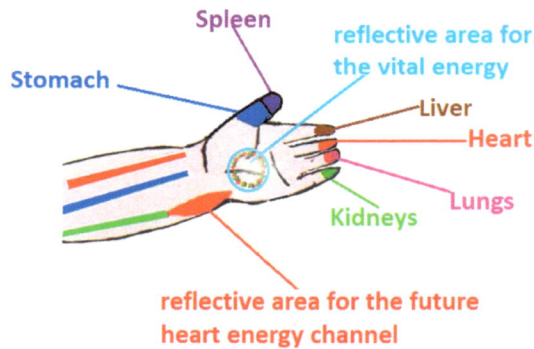

Picture 45. The hand and forehand reflective areas.

5. Calming the back muscles.

The long moves at the back of your kid. You can continue the session with the long reflective moves alongside the spine, pressing gently with your thumbs on the reflective areas related to the shoulders, neck, chest, and lower back muscles marked with green circles. The stimulation of the orange-marked reflective area is beneficial for the prevention of the common cold and upper respiratory tract infections. You can use the red-marked muscle pathways during your reflexology by your kid's bloating, gas ache in the belly and any digestive infirmities, which are very common in kids.

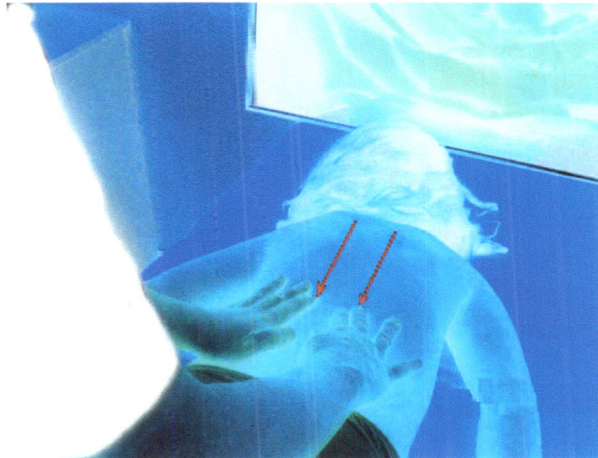

Picture 46. The muscle pathways and reflective areas at the back of your kid.

6. The crown reflexology.

A gentle pressing and rubbing on the top area of your kid's head will send impulses to strengthen the muscles and promote your kid's growth and development. The highest point at the crown of your kid relates to growth and all ligaments and tendons in the kid's body.

7. Grounding the feet.

Apply gentle pressure with your index finger and thumb on the line between the big and second toe. There are in this area the developing entry points to the liver energy channel. pressing on one of the most prominent lymphatic vessels in the foot, where immune cells can often become stagnant. Your reflexology will help to push these cells back into the lymphatic circulation.

Then gently rub the middle point of the sole forefeet to stimulate the area of the future initial point for the kidneys energy channel, which dominates the kids connection to the soil. At the end hold firm for a while your kid's feet with your palms touching the kid's soles.

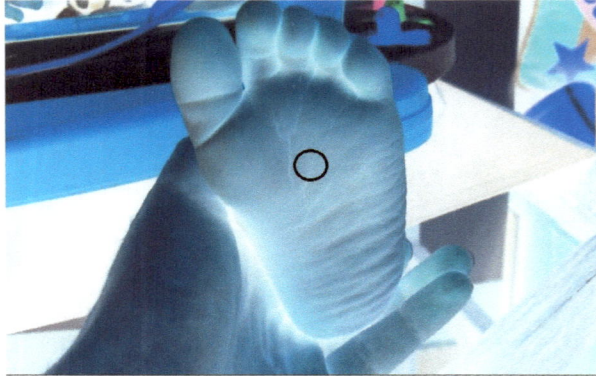

Picture 47. A child's foot. Plantar view. By FA RenLis - Own work. Wikipedia. Modified.

8. Breathing regulation.

A funny reflexology grip can invigorate your kid's breathing. Sometimes, you can experience that your kid, by this reflexology on the reflective area beside the belly, button can be ticklish.

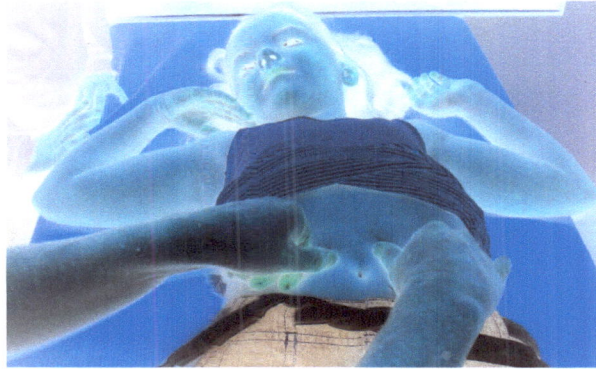

Picture 48. A grip for invigoration of the kid's breathing.

It means your kid is overstimulated with the outer world, school or learning experiences and does not have correct abdominal breathing. Moving to this reflective area and returning to the finger or forearm is the best way to adapt your kid to this extraordinary important, essential area for reflexology.

This structured reflexology, which will last about 20 minutes, is only a guideline. It is entirely up to you to find your own sequence with your kid and apply it in the way your kid likes best. This flexibility empowers you to tailor the practice to your kid's needs and preferences.

~ 14 ~

EAR REFLEXOLOGY

Ear reflexology, also known as auricular therapy, is a gentle and non-invasive form of natural medicine. It operates on the principle that the ear is a mini embryonic representation of the entire body, with each body part, organ, and gland mapped out on the ear. By stimulating specific pressure points around the ear, this technique can effectively release muscles tension and promote general health

The roots of ear reflexology can be traced back to the groundbreaking work of French neurologist Dr Paul Nogier.

In 1958, Dr Nogier discovered the hologram of the embryo in the inverted position, a discovery that revolutionized the field of reflexology and paved the way for auricular therapy as we know it today.

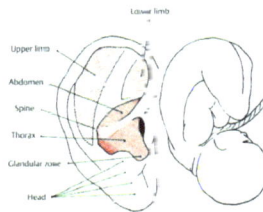

Picture 49. Dr Nogier's embrionic picture in the ear.

Dr. Paul Nogier described his discovery in his book entitled *The Man in the Ear*, published in 1985. His finding of the embryo in the ear is best illustrated through a visual representation. The image above clearly shows how the ear contains a miniaturized representation of the unborn child as it is positioned in the womb, with each body part, organ, and gland mapped onto the ear. Dr. Nogier's auricular acupuncture was introduced to China in 1958.

If you take a closer look, as I did, you will see two embryonic representations in the ear.

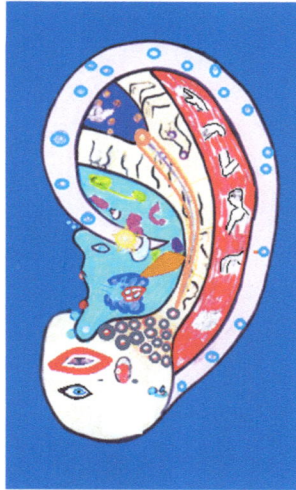

Picture 50. Mini holograms in the ear.

The first representation in the ear mirrors the embryo in the womb, complete with the body's new brain and motoric muscle system. The second, displayed in blue, seems to be an ancient, more animal representation, with the areas representing all internal organs regulated mainly by your subconscious vegetative system.

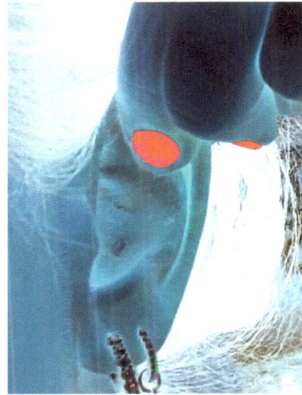

Picture 51. Ear reflexology.

Ear self-reflexology is easy to perform and safe. Pressure on the upper region of the ear has an anti-inflammatory effect and sometime can replace the pain killers. It needs to be exercised several times.

~ 15 ~

REFLEXOLOGY WITH THE FEET

Reflexology, which typically involves touching, rubbing, or kneading the body's soft tissues, takes on a unique form with Ashiatsu massage. In this technique, therapists use their bare feet to apply deep compression, long gliding strokes, and assisted stretching. This approach offers distinct benefits that are worth exploring. Additionally, Ashiatsu is practiced by Shaolin monks at the Shaolin Temple in Henan, China, enhancing its appeal. This remarkable combination of reflexology and massage is particularly beneficial for athletes, as it effectively reduces lower back pain and muscle strain while improving flexibility. It is an interesting method that can increase circulation in clients with thick or muscular builds more rapidly than traditional hands-on reflexology.

Miss Dawn Dotson, a licensed massage practitioner, performs Ashiatsu massages on U.S. Army Corps of Engineers Europe District employees, May 10, 2011, as part of the district's Health Fair. The annual event runs through May 12 and includes CPR and Yoga classes, health assessments and a 5k Fun Run/Walk. U.S. Army Corps of Engineers photo by Carol E. Davis.

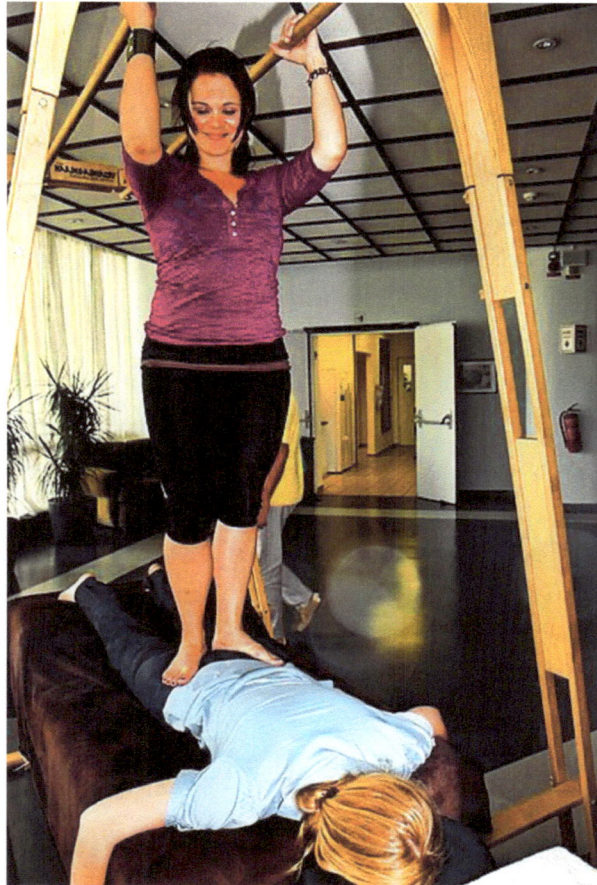

Picture 52. Ashiatsu reflexology performed by the feet by a licensed therapist. Wikipedia.

ABOUT THE AUTHOR

Dr Jerzy (George) Dyczynski, MD, MBA, is a highly experienced physician with a strong interest in modern, conventional, and traditional medical approaches. His career began in 1976 as a medical doctor in the emergency unit of a Cardiology Department in Poland, and has since taken him to various healthcare settings across Germany, Switzerland, China, and Australia, showcasing his adaptability and global perspective.

Dr George is passionate about holistic medicine, particularly holistic heart health, and enjoys helping patients improve their wellness and well-being. With a clinical background as a medical doctor, specialist in internal medicine, and cardiologist, he is equipped to address a wide range of complex conditions, including cardiovascular and stress-related issues.

Drawing on his extensive medical knowledge and professional training, Dr George customizes each treatment plan, integrating evidence-based practices with holistic approaches. His medical tools include modern medicine, acupuncture, specialized breathing and oxygenation techniques, and lifestyle interventions. Over the years, he has performed more than 30,000 acupuncture treatments for various conditions in private practice, a university clinic, and a hospital setting.

Patients describe Dr George as a dedicated doctor, compassionate researcher, and world-class acupuncturist. He values collaboration with his patients, working closely with them to ensure the best outcomes and empowering them to achieve comprehensive health and true wellness in the 21st century.

Dr Jerzy holds a doctorate in Cardiology, a field in which he has made significant contributions through numerous articles in international journals and scientific presentations. He has received qualifications in medical quality management from the Bavarian Medical Council in Munich and earned his medical MBA from the University of Lueneburg in Germany.

For four years, Dr George served as the leading physician and a specialist for internal medicine at a family clinic in the Black Forest region of Germany, where he treated kids using reflexology, while their parents benefited from acupuncture. He supervised four reflexology and massage therapists in that role.

In 2000, he presented a pediatric massage workshop at the World Congress of Natural Medicine in Edmonton, Canada.

Additionally, Dr Jerzy presented his work at the World Congress of Acupuncture on the Gold Coast, Australia, in 2004, alongside his wife Angela, a Quality Manager. Their lecture was quoted as the best presentation of this World Congress of Acupuncture.

Together, they lectured also on foot reflexology at the Australasian Acupuncture and Chinese Medicine Annual Conferences in Melbourne (2005) and Adelaide (2006), demonstrating their expertise in reflexology and traditional medicine.

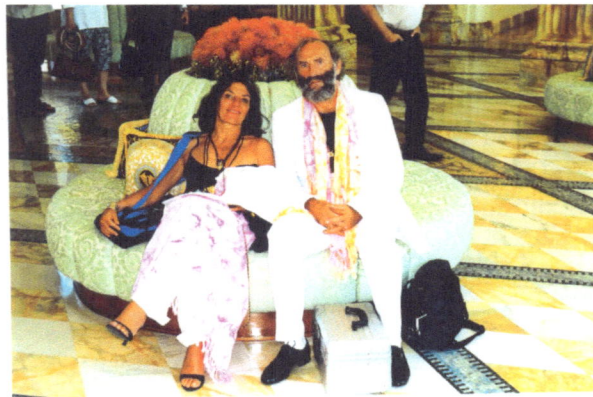

Dr George and Angela during the 6th World Congress of
Acupuncture at Gold Coast, Australia in 2004.

From 2008 to 2009, Dr George worked as a researcher in Heart-Brain Medicine and as a clinical acupuncturist for outpatients at Edith Cowan University Clinic in Perth. His dedication to a holistic approach is a cornerstone of both his professional and personal life. His extensive training in energy channels, traditional gymnastics for health, and over 30 years

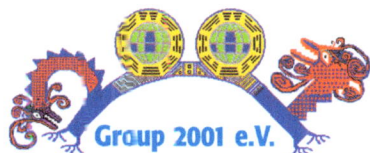

Group 2001 e.V.
for Traditional Chinese Medicine and TCM Infant Massage

Pediatrics Massage Therapy
The precious Pearl of Traditional Chinese Medicine
practical workshop for children parents, therapists and physicians

Pre-Conress August 23-24, 2000, the 4th World Congress of
Medical Acupuncture & Natural Medicine

August, 23, 2000 from 8:00 am - 12:00 noon &
August, 24, 2000 from 1:00 pm - 5:00 pm

The infants hand as a healing gate and a Microsystem
includes the hologram of the whole body.

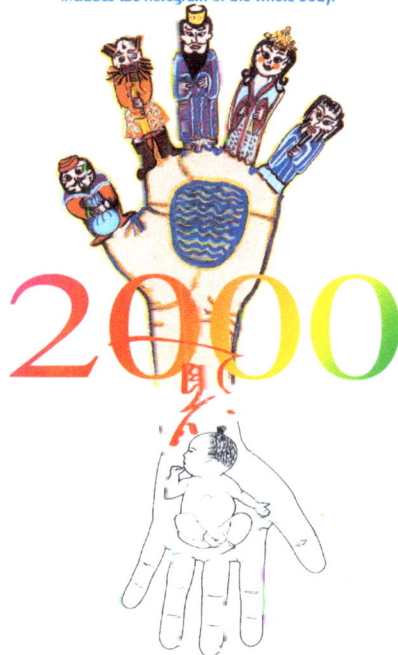

In antient China the five internal organs have been compared to ... organisation of the State
and its government and so -
the middle finger – the Emperor – like the heart
the fourth finger – the Emperors wife – like the lung
the second finger – the Generals – like the liver
the first finger, thumb - Ministry of Finance – like the spleen
the fifth small finger – the Healer or Minister of Science – like the kidney

of kung fu martial arts practice reflect his open-mindedness and his desire to inspire others to explore holistic health.

His most recent works, including "The Dyczynski Program: Healing the Intelligent Heart," published in 2022, and the series Medical Knowledge Made Easy, the first book "Grace in Movement," and the second "Positive Heart Remodeling," published in 2024. This third book, eagerly awaited as a continuation of this successful series, significantly advanced the integration of traditional medicine with its twin modern medicine.

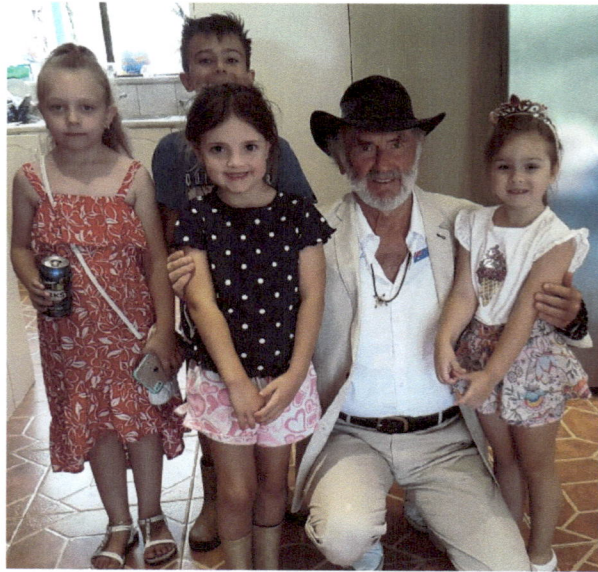

Dr George with country kids in Australia in 2022.

I would like to thank my wife, Angela, and our daughter, Fatima.
They are true co-authors of this book.

www.ingramcontent.com/pod-product-compliance
Lightning Source LLC
Chambersburg PA
CBHW061136030426
42334CB00003B/58